Reiki Healing for Beginners

The Ultimate Masterclass Step-by-Step Guide to Attain Wellness by Unlocking your Chakras, Aura Cleansing, Meditation, Crystals and Self Healing Techniques.

Karen Nhat-Loss

© Copyright 2019 - All rights reserved.

The content contained within this book may not be reproduced, duplicated or transmitted without direct written permission from the author or the publisher.

Under no circumstances will any blame or legal responsibility be held against the publisher, or author, for any damages, reparation, or monetary loss due to the information contained within this book. Either directly or indirectly.

Legal Notice:

This book is copyright protected. This book is only for personal use. You cannot amend, distribute, sell, use, quote or paraphrase any part, or the content within this book, without the consent of the author or publisher.

Disclaimer Notice:

Please note the information contained within this document is for educational and entertainment purposes only. All effort has been executed to present accurate, up to date, and reliable, complete information. No warranties of any kind are declared or implied. Readers acknowledge that the author is not engaging in the rendering of legal, financial, medical or professional advice. The content within this book has been derived from various sources. Please consult a licensed professional before attempting any techniques outlined in this book.

By reading this document, the reader agrees that under no circumstances is the author responsible for any losses, direct or indirect, which are incurred as a result of the use of information contained within this document, including, but not limited to, — errors, omissions, or inaccuracies.

Table of Contents

Introduction 5

Chapter One: Learning Reiki 8

Chapter Two: Advantages of Using Reiki as a System for Healing and Self-Healing 23

Chapter Three: Principles of Reiki 38

Chapter Four: The Power of Attunements 57

Chapter Five: Chakras and Reiki 72

Chapter Six: Reiki Healing and Self-Healing 88

Chapter Seven: Reiki Healing Techniques 105

Chapter Eight: Physical Healing 125

Chapter Nine: Mental, Emotional and Spiritual Healing 143

Chapter Ten: Reiki Level I and II 158

Chapter Eleven: Other Reiki Applications 173

Appendix A 185

Conclusion 187

Introduction

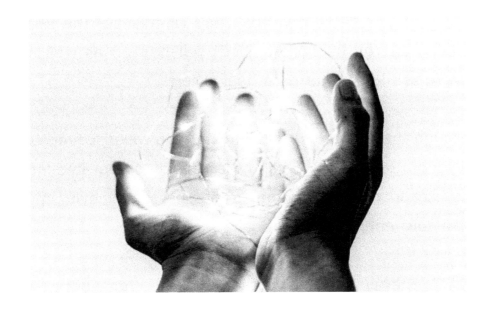

*"The little things? The little moments?
They aren't little."
- Jon Kabat-Zinn*

Congratulations on purchasing your new book, *Reiki Healing for Beginners* and thank you for taking an interest in this series. You will not be disappointed with the knowledge and information contained within these pages.

The following chapters will cover the history of Reiki energy healing, its origins in spiritual study as well as its spread to the western world. They will discuss the uses of Reiki energy healing for both self-healing as well as how to use Reiki energy to heal others.

Through the course of your reading, you will discover the power of Reiki energy and how it can be incorporated into your life in order to increase your personal power and raise your energetic vibration.

Reiki energy is a powerful tool for personal empowerment, mindfulness, and awareness. Through Reiki energy you can achieve physical, emotional, and spiritual health and wellness. Reiki is a unique style of energy work that has been used for centuries in Japan and is a traditional, noninvasive healing modality.

There are plenty of books on this subject on the market, thanks again for choosing this one! Be sure to take a look at the other books in this series *Crystals Healing for Beginners* and *Chakras Healing for Beginners*. All together, these three books complete a series to lead you on the path of empowerment, mindfulness, and personal fulfilment. Every effort was made to ensure it is full of as much useful information as possible, please enjoy!

Chapter One:
Learning Reiki

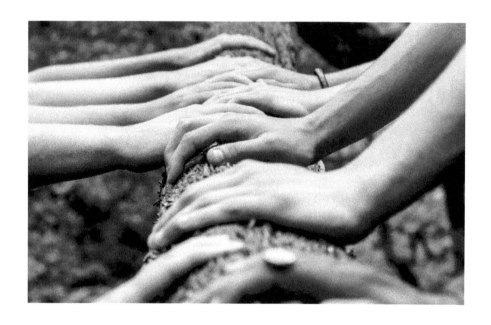

"Everything that has a beginning has an ending. Make your peace with that and all will be well."
- Jack Kornfield

Reiki energy healing is a traditional Japanese healing style. It involves the flow of universal energy as it is channeled through a Reiki practitioner. Reiki is performed with a series of static hand positions that can be placed directly on the body for direct contact or performed hands off, with the hands hovering above the body.

Translated, Reiki is broken into two words. Rei translates into 'Universe' and Ki translates into 'Energy' the same as Qi, or Chi. Reiki means Universal Energy.

The universe is made up of energy. Everything in the universe is made up of energy. Reiki practitioners can connect to that energy on a profound level. Channeling the energy through themselves it can then be used to heal and balance other energetic currents, like the ones found in the human body.

The man most credited for the discovery of Reiki is Dr. Mikao Usui. Dr. Usui grew up in Japan in a family that followed Zen Buddhism traditions. He was born in 1865. After Dr. Usui fell ill during a cholera epidemic, he had a spiritual awakening while he was fighting for his life.

Upon recovering, Dr. Usui went to a Zen monastery where he began his spiritual studies. During his studies, he came across Reiki, a method of healing that had been used for centuries. This healing method used a set of hand positions and symbols that amplified and channeled the energy for healing.

Dr. Usui wanted to use Reiki to heal others, but he felt like he needed more awareness before implementing the healing process. For this awakening he looked inward and started to meditate and practice meditation.

According to legend, as a part of his spiritual journey, he traveled up Mt. Kurama. When he was on the mountain top, he gathered twenty-stones and then he sat down to meditate. For each day that passed on this meditation, Dr. Usui would throw away one of the stones he had gathered. He spent his entire time meditating and studying.

After twenty-one days had passed, Usui opened himself up with the intention of wanting to see things clearly. It was during this time that it is said a bright light flashed above him and rushed towards him. The light beamed through his forehead and Usui saw the Reiki symbols that he had been studying in Sutras at the Zen monastery. It is thought that in this moment, he experienced spiritual enlightenment.

On his travel back down the mountain, legend tells that Usui hurt his foot, and he instinctively placed his hand over his foot, observing that the bleeding stopped and the pain diminished.

Later, Dr. Usui stopped in a village and was given a full meal. He was able to eat the complete meal without any discomfort, despite having been fasting and meditating for twenty-one days. The girl who gave him his meal was experiencing pain and he was able to heal her as well. Upon returning to the monastery, Usui used his healing gift to heal his superior who was suffering from arthritis pain.

Dr. Usui set out on the noble venture of using Reiki to heal the homeless and poor people of Kyoto. He used Reiki in hopes of helping beggars become more productive member of society. Unfortunately, he became discouraged when he found them returning to their habits or begging.

Through this experience, Usui was reminded that it is essential to heal the body, mind, and soul for there to be change. He retreated into meditation again. During this meditation, Usui discovered the five principles of Reiki.

He spent the remainder of his life practicing and teaching Reiki.

In April of 1922, Usui established a Reiki center where he taught Reiki to students and performed sessions for the public.

Traditional Reiki is broken into three levels or degrees of Reiki. The first degree of Reiki is called Shoden (First Degree) and was divided into four levels: Loku-Tou, Go-Tou, Yon-Tou, and San-Tou. The second degree of Reiki is known as Okuden (Inner Teaching) and has two levels: Okuden-Zen-ki (first part) and Okuden-Koe-ki (Second part). The third degree of Reiki is called Shinpiden (Mystery Teaching) and is now called the Master Level.

Chujiro Hayashi was a retired marine and a physician before he began studying Reiki with Usui. As a request from Usui before he died, Hayashi opened his own Reiki clinic to spread the teachings and expand the development of Reiki.

Hayashi kept very meticulous, careful records of the people he treated at his clinic. He kept records of illnesses and conditions and made notes on which Reiki positions and symbols had the best results with various conditions. With his notes and observations, Hayashi wrote Reiki Ryoho Shinshin, which means Guidelines for Reiki Healing Method. He used this guide as a manual in his classes.

In his clinic, Hayashi changed the way Reiki sessions were given and received. He didn't just have clients sit in a chair, but he had them lie on a treatment table. He also began the practice of group sessions where one client would receive simultaneous treatments from several practitioners at once. He developed a new system for giving Reiki Attunements as well.

Hayashi began to change the way Reiki was taught. When he traveled, he would teach the Shoden and Okuden (Reiki degree I and II) together in one seminar that spanned five days. Each day included two or three hours of class instruction as well as one attunement.

Prior to the attack on Pearl Harbor, Hayashi traveled to Hawaii. The Japanese military asked him to report any information on warehouses and military targets in Honolulu. Hayashi refused to make such reports and was thus labeled a traitor by the Japanese government. In

1940, Hayashi performed seppuku (ritual suicide) in order to restore his families honor.

Hawayo Takata is the Reiki Master how is most credited with bringing Reiki to the western world. She also is credited with the growth, development, and expansion of modern Reiki, Reiki teachings, and the spread of Reiki influence.

Takata was born in Hawaii in 1900. Her parents were Japanese immigrants. Takata married a bookkeeper or the plantation where she was also employed. They had two daughters. When her husband died in 1930, Takata had to take on all the labor of her family.

After five years, she began to develop severe abdominal pain and a lung condition. This led to a nervous breakdown. Soon after her breakdown, one of Takata's sisters died and she had to travel to Japan in order to inform her parents who had moved back to their native country.

Takata went into a hospital in Japan for her abdominal pain and the lung condition. She was diagnosed with a tumor and gallstones, asthma, and appendicitis. Rather than getting surgery, Takata went to visit Hayashi's clinic.

Never having experienced Reiki before, Takata was curious, and she was impressed that the diagnosis from the Reiki practitioner was very close to the one she received in the hospital. It was then that Takata began receiving Reiki treatments.

She wanted to learn how to perform Reiki and began to work in Hayashi's clinic and study Reiki. After working in the clinic for a year, she reached her Shinpiden Attunement, Master level.

Takata returned to Hawaii and she began to practice Reiki, opening several clinics. She gave treatments and would teach students up to level II Reiki. She traveled throughout the US and the world, becoming a renowned healer.

After 1970, Takata began teaching students and attuning them to the Master Level, but for a fee of $10,000 for a weekend of training. Usui did not have a high fee for his teachings, and it is speculated that Takata charged a high fee to create respect and credibility for the Reiki discipline.

Takata did not believe that treatments and teachings should be given for free. She did not provide her students with written course material and forbade them from taking notes or recordings. When she taught the Reiki symbols, she made her students memorize them and did not allow them to draw them out or make copies of them.

Traditionally, Reiki was taught orally, and Takata wanted to keep that the traditional teaching method. Although neither Usui or Hayashi stuck to oral traditions. Takata received a Reiki manual from Hayashi during her studies.

Takata changed the way that Reiki was taught by simplifying and refining the hand positions she had been taught.

By the time Takata died in 1980, she had attuned and initiated twenty-two Reiki masters. She made her students promise to keep teaching Reiki the same way that she had taught them.

This teaching avenue made Reiki a rather exclusive organization in both Japan and the US. Over time though, Masters that Takata had trained began to lower their fees. This changed the way Reiki was taught with more of an emphasis on the wisdom of Reiki guiding the sessions.

Reiki classes became more open and accessible. Using workbooks and printed study material came back into practice. Students were encouraged to study under different practitioners and Masters for a more well-rounded learning experience. These shifts allowed for Reiki to become more widely taught. It is estimated that there are now over four million Reiki practitioners in the world and over one million Reiki Masters.

When learning and studying Reiki there are going to be several methods for your learning experience. Some Masters will teach more traditionally, breaking the course up into the three degrees, teaching each level individually. Each level might be a weekend long class experience with additional work to perform on your own before progressing to the next level.

Some Masters might condense all three degrees into one weekend long seminar and then encourage you to continue studying and working on your own to hone your skills. With the spread of technology and online courses that are readily available, some Masters have brought their teachings to online courses.

Sometimes online courses are more practical because you can work at your own pace and don't need to stick to a strict schedule. This means you can work around your own busy lifestyle and still learn. You won't have to take time off or even travel to a Master for a weekend course. Since Reiki can be performed over distances, then doing online course work and then getting your Attunements from a distance, is just as effective.

Some Reiki courses do provide their students with excellent course material for study. Some courses might require students to do continued work outside of the class. A common follow up practice to Reiki Level I could be to perform twenty-one self-healing Reiki session on consecutive days. This is to simulate Usui's twenty-one days of meditation.

After receiving your Reiki Level II attunement, you might be required to perform five consecutive self-treatments, five consecutive treatments on someone else, and five consecutive distance treatments. These treatments should incorporate the Reiki symbols when possible.

Whether you decide to take an online course or study Reiki in an in-person seminar or class setting, make sure to accurately and seriously complete any assignments that are given to you. In order to get the most out of your study, you are going to want to treat it like any other class. If an assignment is to draw out the Reiki symbols on a piece of paper every day for a week, that may seem silly and time consuming, but cutting corners in the coursework won't give you the best learning experience.

Regardless of if you are taking an online course or an in-person course, you should find a Reiki Master that you can talk to, share experiences with, and get sessions from. Maybe they'll even trade sessions with you. This Reiki Master doesn't necessarily have to be the Master that you are learning from in your courses. Having a mentor of sorts will greatly enhance your experience in learning Reiki.

When deciding what kind of course to take, do your research on the Master that is teaching the course. What is their experience level? Do they have good reviews? Do their students have success in their field after the course? Does the course have any kind of standardized testing or take-home work?

You'll want to look for courses that meet your own needs, but you'll also want to find a course that is going to be worth your time and money. Don't be discouraged or turned off to a course just because it is online. Don't think that a course lacks credibility because it teaches Reiki Level I and II in one seminar.

There are so many ways to learn Reiki now. This is both a blessing and a possible curse. You should easily be able to find a course style that fits with your schedule and life. However, since it is so easy for Masters to post a generic online course that they just post PowerPoint presentations for, you'll want to be careful not to get into a course that doesn't have to merit or information that you are seeking.

Usui Reiki is also called Traditional Reiki. This is the Reiki discipline that has the three degrees of Reiki. There are other Reiki traditions that have developed that can have nine degrees to learn. This book is primarily going to cover information that is aligned with Traditional Reiki.

When studying Reiki, it is important to remember that you don't need to learn beyond Reiki Level I if you do not feel called to. Reiki Level II and the Master Level do provide additional tools for Reiki, deepen your connection to Reiki energy, and also offer advanced Reiki Techniques. However, if you are comfortable with Reiki Level I, there may not be a need to progress.

Reiki Attunements last forever, so you only need to receive the Attunements once. Reiki is a skill though and does require practice to keep those skills sharp. There are some cases in which a Reiki Master may ask you to receive additional Attunements. If you took Reiki Level I and then sought a different Master for Reiki Level II, they might require you to receive both Reiki Level I and II attunements from them.

If you studied Reiki eleven years ago and then decided to get back into it, your Master might require you to get the Attunements again if you take a refresher course. While you won't need the Attunements to practice Reiki, it doesn't hurt to get them and help reopen those channels, especially if you haven't actively been practicing Reiki.

You can use Reiki as a self-healing method only, or as a professional healing service to heal paying clients. If you do decide to see clients, it is recommended that you at least progress through Reiki Level II. This isn't required and many Reiki Level I practitioners have successful businesses. Reiki Level II will simply increase your knowledge of Reiki, attune you to the Reiki Symbols, and deepen your wisdom. This can create a more powerful healing experience for yourself and others.

There is no harm in taking a Reiki level I course and then staying at that level until you feel called to progress to the next level. You may never feel called to. It might take months, or years for you to feel like you want to move forward with your studies. Wherever you are comfortable in your spiritual journey is where you should be.

Chapter Two:
Advantages of Using Reiki as a System for Healing and Self-Healing

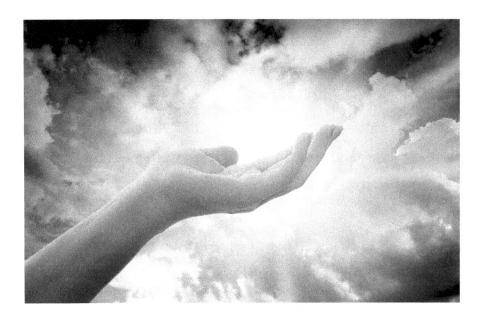

"You cannot control the results, only your actions."
- *Allan Lokos*

There are many bodywork styles that can work well with the physical, energetic, and emotional bodies. Massage therapy, acupuncture, chiropractic adjustments, and reflexology are all well known and have amazing benefits. Reiki is a more unique style of bodywork because it is highly intuitive and doesn't require extensive knowledge of anatomy. With Reiki, you don't intend to target specific parts of the body, Reiki energy goes where it is most needed.

However, there are benefits to knowing the basics of human anatomy and how it relates to different symptoms. Even if you only plan on using Reiki on yourself, understanding the different relationships between key systems in the body, you'll better be able to trace the source of your symptoms.

All symptoms that present in the body, whether it is physical pain, illness, injury, or disease, stem from an energetic imbalance in the body which creates dis-ease. Dis-ease opens the doors and windows for the body to be incapable of functioning at its optimal health and wellness levels. When the body can't function at those levels it begins to experience problems in the body systems which then lead to pain, illness, injury, and disease.

Symptoms of dis-ease can also manifest in an emotional or spiritual way. Many mental health conditions can be a result of dis-ease. As can the manifestation of trauma and anxiety disorders. Obsessive compulsive disorder, attention deficit disorder, nightmares, they can also be results of imbalance and dis-ease in the body.

Using Reiki to treat symptoms of dis-ease will eventually lead back to the root cause. In many cases, knowing the root cause of the dis-ease is only half the battle. Once you've identified a cause within yourself, you may need to take extra steps to change your lifestyle in order to prevent the dis-ease from coming back. Healing comes from within, which is why self-healing is the most effective path towards a more positive, empowered lifestyle.

Again, this is why Reiki is so amazing, because you can use it to heal yourself. During a self-treatment session, you can discover the root cause of your symptoms through the intuitive experiences you have when treating yourself. If you receive Reiki sessions from other practitioners, you may not get the same intuitive information. Your Reiki Practitioner will probably pickup on certain imbalances in you through visions and sensations, but they won't be able to interpret what those visions and sensations mean to you. You will have to discover the meanings for yourself and what you can change in your life to prevent the dis-ease from returning.

When performing Reiki sessions on others, your intuition might guide you to sources of their dis-ease. However, since healing comes from within, you can only guide them in the right direction. You can never interpret what something means to someone else for them. Nor can you tell them the best way to resolve whatever conflicts they are experiencing. This is why self-healing is so important.

Knowing enough basic anatomy on the energetic, physical, and emotional level you can better understand what you feel and what the sources of your own dis-ease is.

Chakras

The chakra system is comprised of seven main chakras that sit along the spine. There are additional sub chakras throughout the body with as many as up to one hundred and fourteen.

Chakra translated from Sanskrit means disk or wheel. Chakras are spinning energetic pools that connect the physical body, the energetic body, and the emotional body. They are the convergence point of the three bodies coming together. They are the centers of energy in the body, with a swirling energy that rotates in both a clockwise and counterclockwise directions.

The chakras are cone shaped. The apex of the cone is right on the spine and then the cone extends outwards in both the front and the back of the body. The two exceptions are the crown chakra which expands up from the top of the head and the root chakra which expands down towards the feet out the tail of the spine.

The seven main chakras are the crown chakra at the top of the head. The third eye chakra at the crown and occiput. The throat chakra at the base of the throat and the top of the shoulder blades. The heart chakra at the center of the sternum and between the shoulder blades on the back. The solar plexus chakra an inch or two above the naval and above the sacrum. The sacral chakra an in or two below the naval and at the sacrum. The root chakra is at the base of the spine.

Each chakra resonates with a body cavity, organs, and organ systems. These chakras also align with emotional and energetic components of the body, mind, and spirit. This is how energetic imbalances and dis-ease can then contribute to manifestations of illness, disease, injury, and emotional conditions and disorders. Since the chakras are so connected to different layers of the body, they can be a source of imbalance that presents moderate to severe symptoms.

Reiki is a balancing healing modality. It resonates well with the chakras and helps to realign their energies, thus resulting in fewer symptoms and a healthier life. How Reiki can be used with and benefit the chakras is going to be elaborated on in future chapters. Another book in this series *Chakras Healing for Beginners* is another source of how the chakras and Reiki energy work together.

Chakras are a well-known part of the energetic anatomy and the physical anatomy. There are plenty of ways to balance and heal the chakras. One of the benefits of Reiki is that Reiki can be sent over time and space. It can be used to heal deeply rooted past traumas that may have been repressed, or even forgotten about. These traumas never fully go away, but might become overshadowed by the manifestation of more prevalent or current symptoms. Imbalances that go unaddressed can end up in a much different place than where they started.

Aura

The aura is another commonly known energetic system that is part of the body. Think of your aura like a personal bubble. The concept of the personal bubble derives from the aura. The aura is an electromagnetic energy frequency that is projected by your individual energetic vibration.

The aura can be expanded out away from the body or retracted to be closer to the body. The health of your aura is going to contribute to your physical, mental, and emotional health as well. Your aura is in a sense, a shield for you and energies around you. It can protect you from unwanted energies, but if it is unhealthy or imbalanced this protection is greatly diminished.

The aura is also a tool for you to attract people and situations in your life that resonate with your personal energy. Energies attract and repel each other. If your aura is raised to the energetic frequency that you most strongly align with, then other people, jobs, and life situations that are going to compliment you and your personal power.

Around your body, the aura exists in seven layers. Each layer corresponds to one of the seven main chakras. The first layer of the aura is about 1-2 inches from the body and resonates with the root chakra. The second auric layer is roughly 3-4 inches from the body and correlates to the sacral chakra. The third layer of the aura sits 5-6 inches from the body and it is related to the solar plexus chakra. The fourth auric layer is between 7-8 inches from the body and it resonates with the heart chakra.

The fifth layer of the aura is the pastel color layer. It relates to the throat chakra and is about 9-10 inches from the body. This is the colored layer that can be seen as a reflection of your personal energetic vibration. The sixth layer of the aura resonates with the third eye chakra and rests between 11 and 12 inches from the body. It is a silver light layer that is a shield for you against unwanted and negative energies. The seventh aura later is about 13-14 inches from the body and correlates to the crown chakra. The seventh layer is comprised of beads. These beads can become cracked or damaged over time due to exposure to all the energies in the world. The beads wear down over time and need to be refreshed.

Reiki energy healing is a wonderful form of energy that helps balance the aura. It realigns the layers with the chakras and rejuvenates your personal protective bubble.

Lymphatic System

The lymphatic system is one of the main components of the immune system. Comprised of lymphatic vessels, lymphatic ducts and lymph nodes. Lymph is a fluid that runs through the lymphatic vessels and helps remove waste from the body, organs, and organ systems.

The thoracic duct in the chest is the main vessel of the lymphatic system. Unlike the circulatory system that has the heart to pump blood through your veins, the lymphatic system requires bodily movement to keep lymph flowing properly.

This is one reason that exercise and movement is so important to the health of the body. Without it, lymph doesn't flow properly. This leads to blockages in the system. It also leads to improper cleaning of the body and deteriorates the functionality of the immune system.

Overtime this leads to many issues in the body on a physical, mental, and spiritual level. It can be hard to trace these blocks back to the lymphatic system, especially because they are physical blocks, not necessarily energetic blocks. An energetic imbalance in one of the chakras can lead to a lack of motivation or energy which results in a lack of movement and exercise, thus becoming an issue with the lymphatic system.

Reiki is a subtle energy. It is noninvasive. Yet it stimulates the energetic currents in the body, like the nervous system electrical impulses. It can balance the chakras that link to motivation and energy, which can provide you with the personal power to begin moving and exercising, even if it is just for a twenty minute walk every day.

The lymphatic system is a part of the physical anatomy, but it has strong ties to the energetic anatomy. Since it is a part of the immune system and without proper energetic balance, the immune system weakens, the two together are closely entwined. This correlation is another reason that Reiki energy is such a powerful healing tool for the lymphatic system.

The thoracic duct of the lymphatic system closely resonates with the heart chakra and can be stimulated by the static hand positions of a Reiki treatment placed over the heart chakra. When combined with other healing methods such as crystals, this can enhance the focus of Reiki energy specifically on the heart chakra or the thoracic duct. Even though Reiki is intuitive by nature, it can be focused with the implementation of other healing methods like crystals.

Muscular System
Muscles in the body are a source of structure, movement, and strength. Muscles move the bones and joints which move the limbs. Muscles move the mouth to assist with speech and facial expressions.

Movement is a source of energy in the body. If the muscles are imbalanced, then this can result in a lack of movement and a lack of energy flow in the body. The muscular system is controlled by electrical impulses from the nervous system. Electricity is another form of energetic current in the body.

Muscles, ligaments, and tendons are all part of the muscular system. Fascia connective tissue is part of the muscular system.

The muscular system can also become a major source of pain and discomfort in the body. Muscular pain is some of the hardest to diagnose unless there is a torn or ripped tendon, ligament or muscle. There are over six hundred muscles in the human body. Determining what exact muscle is the source of pain and then what is causing that pain can become quite difficult. MRI's and X-rays only do so much when looking at the muscular system.

When it comes to connective tissue like fascia, a lot of the information on fascia is still new and surfacing in the medical community. Conditions such as plantar fasciitis have been somewhat controversial in the past.

The muscles have such a connection with different energetic currents in the body, it is no wonder that Reiki energy healing can balance and benefit the muscles so profoundly. Reiki interacts with the kinetic energy, potential energy, and the electrical energy of the muscles. When there is an energetic imbalance this means that there can be an overactivity in energy or a block somewhere in the system.

Fortunately, with Reiki, you do not need to know if there is a block or an overactivity in order for Reiki to heal the imbalance. Different symptoms might present for a block as for overactive energy. With Reiki, you don't need to know the nature of the imbalance because Reiki intuitively goes where it is needed and works on the energetic imbalances. It might take several sessions for you to experience relief or notice changes in the imbalances. Sometimes, the results are so subtle, you might not notice them right away.

With the muscular system, imbalances often lead to pain and injury, so the results of Reiki healing may be more noticeable.

Endocrine Systems

When it comes to functionality of the body, the endocrine system is one of the most important systems. The endocrine system includes glands and controls the production and excretion of hormones and enzymes. Hormones control homeostasis in the body. Hormones assist with sexuality, fertility, and even emotional responses. Enzymes assist with digestion and other functions in the body.

The thyroid gland, adrenal glands, ovaries, salivary glands, testis, pituitary glands, and all the other glands in the body are a part of the endocrine system. These glands produce and excrete the hormones and enzymes that contribute to the balance in your body.

Anyone who has had a hormone disorder, or a problem with their thyroid gland, or even severe mood swings during menstruation have had experiences with severe hormonal imbalances.

The chakras correlate with specific glands and their hormones. This means that an energetic imbalance in the chakras can lead to a gland or hormone disorder or disease. Reiki energy balances those chakras and keeps the endocrine system balanced, producing hormones and enzymes appropriately.

The body can be thrown completely out of functioning parameters if the endocrine system isn't working. The immune system can fail, fertility problems can arise, lack of sexual interest or libido, and emotional problems can result. Other issues such as the inability to make decisions and not being able to think rationally are also impacted by the endocrine system.

It is important to keep the endocrine system producing and secreting hormones and enzymes within balance. Reiki energy healing can correct imbalances and bring the endocrine system back into alignment leading to a healthy body, mind, and spirit.

Chapter Three:
Principles of Reiki

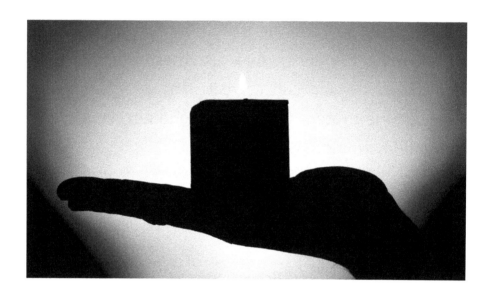

"If the problem can be solved, why worry? If the problem can't be solved, worrying will do you no good."
- Buddha

Reiki operates on Five Principles that Dr. Usui discovered in his meditation practices. These five principles are a way to release the stories and energies that your mind tells you that create suffering in your daily life.

Generally, daily activities aren't meant to cause stress and anxiety. It is the mind and the beliefs that stay in the mind which create that stress and anxiety. My unraveling those limitations, your mind can let go and you can have a sense of balance and peace in your life and in your thoughts.

These five principles allow you to improve your actions and thought patterns day to day and moment by moment. Your conscious thoughts and actions over time become your natural way of thinking and being. That is the importance of the five Reiki principles.

The five Reiki principles are:

- For all of today, I will not worry
- For all of today, I will not be angry
- For all of today, I will work honestly
- For all of today, I will be grateful for my blessings
- For all of today, I will be kind to all living things

These principles can become important in your everyday life. To incorporate the principles, into your life, you can say them aloud like mantras. You can use them in your daily meditations, or write them out and post them on a wall, or at your desk at work.

Each individual feels a different resonance with the five principles and will gain a different meaning from them. These meanings and resonances can change over time. When you first start working with these principles, they might carry a certain resonance, and then over time they might begin to mean something new to you.

If the traditional principles in Reiki don't resonate with you, trying different wording. Some other popular variations include:

- Just for today, I will trust
- Just for today, I will love
- Just for today, I will be true to myself and others
- Just for today, I will give thanks for my blessings
- Just for today I will be kind to every living thing

Another practice for getting in touch with these principles and making them a part of your life is to hold their intention and really feel what it feels like. You can meditate and focus on the principles while lying down or sitting up.

Try closing your eyes and repeating each of the principles out loud, several times. You can also practice saying them in your mind and use whatever method feels the most comfortable. Take the time to sit with each principle and really feel its intention and its meaning wash over you and through you.

As you perform these exercises with the five Reiki principles, you might want to document the different experiences, feelings, and sensations that come up for you. Keeping a journal can help you see your personal growth and progression with the Reiki principles as you keep including them into your healing and your life.

For all of today, I will not worry
Worry as an emotion can be helpful. Worry can help work through some situations in a healthy way. When worry occurs in excess or occurs frequently, it can become problematic. Anytime an emotion becomes problematic it impacts the body, mind, and spirit.

When you worry, your mind is focused on the future. Although a small amount of worry can be helpful in taking action in the present, excessive worry can lead to anxiety, confusion, and stagnation. Being present in the moment is how you can be most effective. Through this principle, you will learn to trust in the wisdom of Reiki to guide you through life's ups and downs.

When you experience difficulty, those moments often leave to the most crucial points of development. Developing a fearful and worrisome mindset you will begin to see positive and neutral events only from a negative perspective. Releasing those beliefs will instead help you perceive situations from a more positive angle.

Be open to where life is leading you and enjoy the ride that is life. Life gives you ups and downs, be present for it all to empower yourself for growth and change. To really support this Reiki principle, make time in your day for activities that you enjoy. Surround yourself with people who resonate with a peaceful, happy energy. That energy will become a part of you as well.

For all of today, I will not be angry
The emotion of anger stems from a place where you feel like you have no control or a lack of power. When a perceived negative event occurs that you have a strong association with, the emotion may not be processed

properly or released. The body stores the emotion rather than releasing it. When another even occurs that reminds you of the original event that anger resurfaces from where it was stored, only this time you have anger that is responding to both evens and is stronger, causing heightened reactions.

Over time, the emotions get stored up more and more, creating pressure. Then a simple trigger can result in an explosive reaction.

Part of working with Reiki energy and in healing yourself is in processing and releasing stored emotions in a constructive, healthy way. Anger is difficult to process in a healthy way because society teaches people from a young age that anger is negative and shouldn't be expressed.

If you experience anger, take a step back from the situation, then breathe into the anger. Become a witness to the even. From the viewpoint of being a witness you will be able to let that anger emotion pass through you rather than storing it for a later event.

Meditating on a daily basis on what the absence of anger feels like can help you process this emotion more effectively. Additionally, if you meditate on choosing to feel emotions that are a higher vibration than anger, you can help yourself default to more positive thought patterns rather than storing the anger.

When angry, taking deep breath after deep breath, and focusing on those breaths, can actually help you feel the release of the pressure that is built up from anger. Every person and every experience have a lesson for you. Approaching situations and people from a place of wanting to learn and being open to knowledge, you'll find that these lessons come easier. Responding to an event or a person in anger results in an incomplete lesson and you are more likely to relive that event with more intense energies and emotions.

For all of today, I will work honestly
In your heart of hearts, you know when you are being honest with yourself. When you aren't being honest, dissatisfaction becomes your body's way of showing you that you aren't being honest.

By not honoring your own dreams, passions, and talents, you lead a dishonest life. If you make decisions based on fear then you are definitely not being true to your soul or your heart.

The role you have to play is very important in this world. The role that each individual has to play in this world is important. The way you live and your actions make a difference in the lives of everyone that crosses your path. Assuming you don't have that impact does not serve yourself or the world. The impact you are here to make is guided by your dreams and desires. This helps you discover what the universe wants for you to accomplish. Honor yourself by following your dreams and live honestly.

For all of today, I will be grateful for my blessings
It is not uncommon to view events as good or bad. This is a result of the ego getting in the way. The soul or spirit, however, sees each event as an opportunity to grow and strengthen. Each experience brings you to a place that you can increase your awareness, and mindfulness.

Many people continue to search for external sources of pleasure, happiness, and gratification. It is the hope that these external sources will make you feel good and the mentality of 'I will be happy when...' becomes a thought at the forefront of the mind. It can be a hard lesson to learn that the true source of happiness comes from within.

You can start learning this and experiencing this by being grateful for your blessings every day. Be grateful now, in this moment, at this time and it will bring more positivity into your life. As you project this gratefulness and experience it, your environment will shift to match those changes.

Gratitude is a powerful intention. Gratitude raises the vibration of your body, mind, and spirit as well as bringing you insight and wisdom. Everyone, including you, has countless things to be grateful for. Defaulting to this Reiki principle is going to help you focus on your blessings and allow you to bring much more into your life.

Holding the intention of gratitude every day will have a dramatic effect on your life. You can even use Reiki to hold that intention of gratitude as well as one of the Three

Pillars of Reiki, the Gassho, which will be discussed further along in this chapter.

When using Reiki to hold your intention of gratitude, you can place one hand on your third eye chakra at your brow and the other on the third eye chakra at the base of your skull.

For all of today, I will be kind to all living things
As previously touched on, the energetic frequency that you project or emanate will attract other things, people, jobs, and situations, that also resonate with that energy. Holding a high vibration will bring you to people and situations with similar high vibrations.

There is a study by Dr. Masuro Emoto where he researches the results of intentions with water. Negative intentions, like spoken words and thoughts, changed the molecular composition of the water in a less than appealing way. This was photographed at a molecular level to display the differences in how water exposed to negative intentions differed from water exposed to positive intentions.

The human body is made up of eighty percent water. Focusing on intentions such as kindness and positivity stand to change your water composition on a molecular level and increase your energetic vibration. It keeps the body, mind, and spirit, healthy. The individuals that you encounter every day serve as mirrors into yourself. By keeping your energetic vibration high, the people you interact with start to reflect that as well.

It is your choice to life a life of peace, balance, and satisfaction. You have the power to create that life for yourself. Why pass that up?

Even Dr. Usui who discovered and performed Reiki, spent a great deal of his time in meditation and inner contemplation for personal and spiritual growth. He worked to increase his awareness to become a strong and effective conduit to channel Reiki energy through himself. Along with incorporating the five Reiki principles into your life and mentality, performing Reiki treatments on yourself every day will also make a difference. Release the limiting beliefs imposed on you by society and that you've put on yourself and your own world.

Along with the five Reiki principles, there are Three Pillars of Reiki that are going to improve your life, your vibration, and your environment. They will also help you connect more deeply with Reiki energy and healing.

The Three Pillars of Reiki are:

- Gassho (Gash-Show)
- Reiji-Ho (Ray-Gee-Hoe)
- Chiryo (Chi-Rye-Oh)

These three Reiki pillars are going to help deepen your connection to Reiki energy. They are going to aid you in your work with the five Reiki Principles. More than that they are going to provide you with additional tools to help in your self-treatment sessions and with the work you do with clients.

The three Reiki Pillars are taught in the Reiki Level II course because they do include some more advanced techniques and sometimes employ the use of Reiki Symbols which are taught at Reiki Level II. However, you can adapt them and find ways to include them into your every day healing and Reiki practice without using the advanced Reiki symbols.

Gassho

Gassho is a type of Reiki meditation. The translation of Gassho is: two hands coming together. The Gassho meditation is meant to hold the intention of gratitude, focus, respect, connection, and balance to collective consciousness.

Dr. Usui's students were taught to place their hands in the Gassho position each morning and each night. Gassho helps to quiet and focus the mind during meditation. It can be incorporated into a meditation or be what you use to start your meditation to help you focus your mind.

The Gassho position is placing your hands palms together in the prayer position. Close your eyes and bring your awareness to the tips of your middle fingers. Any time your mind begins to wander, gently press your middle fingers together and allow the pressure to help you refocus your intention.

Traditionally, there are two different forms of Gassho. There is formal and informal. Formal Gassho is most commonly used in rituals such as religious services or formal gatherings. Formal Gassho is when you bring your hands together in the prayer position with your fingers pointing towards the sky. Your elbows should be raised with your forearms at an approximately 30-degree angle to the floor. Your fingertips should be level with your eyebrows but your hands should be around four inches from the tip of your nose. Focus your eyes on the tips of your middle fingers.

Mu-shin, which means No Mind, Gassho is a form of Gassho that is used for the purpose of greeting others. In this Gassho meditation, your hands are held together in the prayer position, however you'll want your fingers toughing with a little space between your palms. You'll want your elbows at a 45-degree angle to the floor and your hands four inches from the front of your face. Your fingertips should be just below your nose, lower than the formal Gassho. You can also perform Mu-shin Gassho with your hands positioned in front of the chest above the heart. Again, your eyes should be focused on the tips of your middle fingers.

The recommended amount of time for this meditation is to perform it for about fifteen to thirty minutes. If you find it beneficial, try doing this meditation each morning and each evening for a month. Take notes your experiences with Gassho and any changes you notice in your life.

The Gassho meditation should be performed while seated. Whenever a thought or emotion arises, watch them go by and pass through you, continuing on their way and refocus on your fingertips.

Some people find it beneficial to recite the five Reiki principles during a Gassho meditation. If your arms become uncomfortable, lower them down slightly, or put your hands in your lap. When you finish the meditation, send an intention of gratitude. If you need grounding, set your palms on the floor in front of you to end the session completely.

Reiji-Ho

The word Reiji in English means: indication of the Reiki energy. The word Ho means: technique. The Reiji-Ho pillar consists of three techniques that can be performed before each Reiki session. These can help with self-treatment sessions or sessions that are performed on others.

The three rituals of Reiji-Ho are going to align you more deeply with Reiki before you begin channeling it through your body. They are going to enhance each session that you give to yourself or perform on someone else by providing a more focused session.

Step One

The first step in Reiji-Ho is to hold your hands in the Gassho position in front of your chest, eyes closed.

Using the CKR and HSZSN Reiki symbols, ask for the Reiki energy to flow through you. If you do not know the Reiki symbols yet, in your mind, set the strong intention and desire calling on the Reiki energy to flow through you.

Repeat this request three times to shift your mind into that state.

If you are attuned to Reiki Level II, intone the CKR and SHK symbol to hold your intention. If you are not yet attuned to Reiki Level II, assert in your mind that you are holding that intention of Reiki energy flowing through you firmly in your mind.

Step Two

The first part to step two of Reiji-Ho is to ask for the balancing of your client/recipient, or yourself.

Next, you'll want to raise your hands to your third eye chakra at your brow while continuing to keep your hands in the Gassho position.

Set the intention that the Reiki energy will guide your hands to where Reiki energy is needed.

Step Three

Allow the Reiji-Ho technique to guide your hands. Allow your mind to detach from any desires or outcomes regarding the Reiki session you are about to perform. Open yourself up to receiving messages that will help guide you during the session.

Let your hands move over your body or the body of your client. Let your intuition and Reiki guide you to where Reiki is needed. Once Reiji-Ho is complete, your hands will rest.

Place your hands back in the Gassho position again. Then proceed with the Reiki session as normal with hand positions.

It is up to your personal preference whether to discuss anything you find or see during a Reiki session with your clients or recipients.

Chiryo

The word Chiryo means: treatment. To perform Chiryo, you as the practitioner will place your dominant hand over your client's crown chakra. You can also perform Chiryo on yourself by placing your dominant hand over your own crown chakra during a self-treatment.

When you receive an intuitive indication that you should move your hands, begin to move your non-dominant hand over your body or your recipient's body. Allow your hand to follow the guidance you receive from the Reiki energy and your own intuition.

You'll want to keep placing your hands on the body as you are called, holding a position for as long as you are guided to. Chiryo can be performed as a treatment session on its own or as an added aspect to a Reiki session with the traditional hand positions.

Chapter Four:

The Power of Attunements

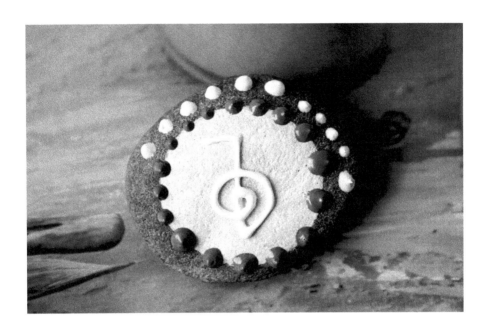

"The mind is like a muscle- the more you exercise it, the stronger it gets and the more it can expand."
- Idowu Koyenikan

Before you can begin practicing Reiki on yourself and others, you'll need to go through a Reiki Attunement process. Each level of Reiki you learn is going to have additional attunements to open you up to different aspects of Reiki. For example, the Reiki Symbols are part of the Reiki Level II attunement process.

Reiki Attunements are the process in which a Reiki Master opens you up to become a channel for the universal energy. Once you receive an attunement, you are forever going to be a channel for Reiki energy, however, the way you live your life is going to be a part of keeping yourself a clear and open conduit for Reiki energy.

You can go years without every practicing Reiki and still retain the attunement. Some people who go long periods of time without practicing Reiki might find that they benefit from receiving an attunement to help clear themselves out and reconnect them Reiki energy. It is not necessary, though.

The Reiki Level I attunement is going to be your first step into using Reiki on yourself and others. The Level I attunement ceremony consists of four attunements that each correspond to one of the four degrees of Reiki Level I. The ceremony includes all four Level I attunements that you can receive during your Reiki Level I course, or at the end of your Reiki Level I course.

A Reiki Level II attunement ceremony is the process that opens you up to the Reiki power symbols. There are three symbols that Dr. Usui discovered and that are part of the Reiki Level II attunement ceremony. This ceremony will be slightly different from the Reiki Level I attunement ceremony because it opens you to a different type of Reiki energy.

The attunement ceremony for the Master Level of Reiki is going to attune you to the Master Reiki Symbol. This symbol is not one of the original power symbols that Dr. Usui used and is only attuned during a Master Level attunement ceremony. This Master attunement ceremony also gives you the knowledge and Reiki wisdom to teach and attune students to Reiki Levels as well.

There are additional attunements for advanced Reiki techniques such as for Crystal Reiki and even Reiki for Animals.

The goal of a Reiki attunement is to clear your body, mind, and spirit of any dissonant energy to ensure that you become a clear conduit for Reiki.

Before the Attunement

Prior to receiving any of your attunements, there are some steps you can take to prepare. While the steps of preparation are optional, it will enhance your experience through your studies and also make the attunements more enjoyable and powerful.

In the twenty-four hours before your attunement ceremony, try to avoid any drug use, recreational and pharmaceutical if possible, and alcohol consumption. Any mind-altering substances or medications that change the chemical composition of your mind or body can hide the true beliefs that cause your suffering.

By abstaining from such substances, you can clear the mind and body to be more alert to your own senses, perceptions, and thoughts. This will greatly enhance your attunement ceremonies and make you a more effective conduit for Reiki energy.

Important note: If you are taking prescribed medications by a medical professional for any kind of condition or treatment of a disease or illness, please keep taking those medications unless your

doctor or medical professional says it is okay to abstain for twenty-four hours.

Another good step to take for the attunement ceremony is to adjust your diet for the twenty-four hours before an attunement and after an attunement. Try to consume only whole, clean foods in that time. Whole, clean foods include legumes, fresh fruits, and vegetables.

Highly processed foods, chemically altered foods, and foods that are covered in preservatives can create blocks in the channels just like alcohol and drugs. By cleansing the body with clean, whole foods that are raw, unprocessed, and healthy will help open up the energetic channels in your body for the attunement ceremony. By continuing that diet for twenty-four hours after receiving the attunement will help you fully feel the effects of your attunement and your connection to Reiki.

By removing any kind of crutch that the body gains from alcohol, drugs, and unclean foods, you have the opportunity to release the stored energy and beliefs that are fed by and supported by those crutches. Those beliefs, memories, and energy stores don't serve your highest self, so releasing them before an attunement is recommended.

For up to a week prior to your attunement, meditating every day leading up to the attunement ceremony and then every day for a week after the ceremony is also going to be helpful. It is recommended that you make mediation a regular part of your daily routine, and practicing that before and after the attunement ceremony can help you to develop that habit.

This mediation process can help you to make the shifts and changes in your life that you hope to sustain with your study of Reiki. After receiving your attunement, you can include a self-treatment session in with your meditation practice as a part of your daily routine.

Reiki Attunement
A Reiki attunement ceremony is performed by a Reiki Master. The Reiki Master performs a routine that includes the Reiki symbols that were discovered by Dr. Usui. During the ceremony, an intention is set for the highest good of the student, the person receiving the attunement.

The Reiki Master will set an intention to strengthen the student's connection to Reiki energy.

Think of the energies in your body like radio waves or radio stations. By changing the radio station, you can change what information you are receiving, such as news, music, the genre of music, talk shows, etc. Just like you can change a radio station to receive different information, you can retune, or reprogram the body to receive different information, like Reiki energy and wisdom.

Without an attunement ceremony, your body does have access to Reiki energy. Everyone's body has access to Reiki energy. It is a part of the universe and a part of being human. Getting attuned to Reiki energy ensures that you as a student and practitioner receive the proper energy signal for Reiki.

A Reiki attunement ceremony takes about twenty to thirty minutes. As the student or recipient of a Reiki ceremony, all you need to do is find a quiet, relaxed space where you will be undisturbed for the course of the ceremony. Just like when you meditate, you may want to play some calming music, have dim lighting and candles, or burn some incense.

Depending on the type of course you take, you might receive your Reiki attunements in person or from a distance. Both are powerful and acceptable methods for receiving and attunement. If you are taking an in-person class and you receive your attunement from your Reiki Master in person, they may have you sit in a chair so they can move around you with ease during the attunement ceremony.

It is recommended that during a Reiki attunement ceremony, you turn off phones, computers, and find a location that is away from sources of the internet and heavy electronic presences. Since Reiki is energy it can come into conflict with other strong energy sources which come from electronics and the internet. In person attunements are generally performed in complete silence.

Whether you are receiving an attunement in person or from a distance, you may have some interesting experiences, like images and sensations. Some students fall asleep during their attunement ceremonies, this isn't uncommon. Other students don't notice anything at all, just feel relaxed. Everyone experiences attunements differently. There is no right or wrong way to experience a Reiki attunement ceremony.

Some common experiences that people have include are varying sensations like hot, cold, or tingling. You could get visions and see images, or even smell or hear things that are a result of Reiki energy.

Some courses of study will perform attunement ceremonies for all three levels of Reiki at once. Other courses will separate the attunement ceremonies out for each level that the student completes.

As with the experiences you have during your attunement ceremony, there is no right or wrong way to receive them.

Each attunement releases dissonant energy from within you and returns your body, mind, and spirit to a natural energetic frequency that your body wants to remain aligned with.

Receiving a Reiki Level I attunement gives you the basics to treat yourself with Reiki and others with Reiki. It is recommended that go through at least Reiki Level II if you'd like to work on clients or recipients, especially in a professional setting.

Going through the Reiki Level II attunement ceremony and the Reiki Master attunement ceremony your body will draw in yet another kind of Reiki energy which is what attunes you to the Reiki symbols and gives you the wisdom to perform attunement ceremonies.

During a ceremony, nothing is actually shifting in your mind, body or spirit. Rather Reiki provides you with a guidance down a path to make shifts that serve your highest good. Your body begins to release, but it is in the inclusion of daily self-treatments after your attunements that push the healing forward and continue to aid you.

Most people that are interested in learning Reiki are ready to release and heal by the time they make the commitment to become a Reiki student. The practice of separating the attunements out was traditionally used in order to ensure that a student was committed to going through each level without rushing the process.

Rushing the attunement ceremonies can result in the student not learning or practicing to the full extent of each level before moving on. Additionally, some students might go through one attunement and then decide that Reiki is for them.

There are times when the energetic shifts happen after an attunement almost immediately. Other times the shifts can take time, practice, and study to occur. The mind puts limitations on itself, especially if you hear a limitation aloud. If a Reiki Master says 'You can't handle more than one Reiki Level Attunement at once,' then the mind imposes that limitation. However, there is no evidence to suggest that attunements can't be performed in one ceremony.

Whatever the case, you should look for a Master who offers the attunement ceremonies in the way that you wish to receive them.

After the Attunement
It isn't uncommon to feel the flow of Reiki energy through your body immediately following an attunement ceremony. If you don't sense energy right away, that is

okay. That doesn't mean there is something wrong with you. It doesn't mean that the attunement didn't work.

Your body is only able to perceive a fraction of energy at any given time, yet the universe is full of energy and anything made of matter is made of energy. It can take time for your body to adjust its perception of Reiki energy.

Your body may begin to change in other ways. Your hands might feel warmer, or tingle and emanate energy when you are around people that are in need of Reiki energy. You'll have to learn to adjust to these sensations. Overtime, you may experience different sensations or shifts in the energy.

If any of the sensations are uncomfortable or overwhelming, take a few deep breaths and set an intention in your mind to allow the Reiki to flow freely through you. This will help release the buildup of intense energy. With practice on yourself, you will begin to learn how to channel the flow of energy and when and how to restrict the flow.

Your body, mind, and spirit will begin to release energy and clear energy. Imbalances will start to be brought back into alignment. Stagnation starts to move and flow again. Any energies that are no longer serving your highest good are transmuted and shifted. These shifts are important to your personal healing, but also to your ability to channel Reiki energy at the highest frequency.

In order to heal, your body must be clear of imbalances. Energetic imbalances are what create dis-ease and lead to the manifestation of physical, emotional, and mental symptoms. After a Reiki attunement ceremony, your body has the wisdom to heal itself. Continuing to promote energy shifts and keeping yourself a clear conduit is what is going to make the largest impact on your personal healing and the raising of your energetic vibration.

You might want to keep track of any changes that you notice occurring. Sometimes having a documented progression of shifts and changes can really help you understand how you are benefitting. If you'd like to use Reiki as a service to help heal others, providing them with personal experiences can help on their road to healing as well.

Once you are attuned to Reiki, it is very important to perform daily self-treatments of Reiki. This is going to keep your body open to Reiki energy and guidance as well as continue to correct any imbalances in your body. Those imbalances will then extend outward into your environment and the lifestyle you live. It is also the best way to keep your body infused with Reiki energy for long-term success and fulfilment.

Drinking adequate amounts of water and keeping your diet as whole and clean as possible are also methods that will help you gain more sensitivity and awareness to energies around you. These are also health practices that will only contribute to your overall health and wellness.

Since Reiki is intuitive, you will need to trust Reiki to heal what needs to be healed. As you perform self-treatments you will begin to understand what this means. That is another reason it is so important to keep up with daily self-treatments once you are attuned.

Reiki Attunements are the ceremonies that are going to open you up to the healing power of Reiki, the wisdom of the universe, and the guiding hand of Reiki energy. When you are ready to receive your attunements and go through the Reiki Level I course, if you have not already done so, be sure to find a Reiki Master that you resonate with and feel like you can learn from.

When you are working closely with someone who is going to be tuning your energy frequencies and guiding you on the attunement journey, you'll want someone you trust. You'll want a Reiki Master that can answer your questions, isn't too busy to make time for their students outside of their set courses, and someone who understands your goals with learning Reiki. Having the right Reiki Master to perform your attunement ceremonies is just as important to your healing journey.

Attunement ceremonies should be enjoyable. It is rare that anyone doesn't enjoy the attunement ceremony, but go into the ceremony with an open mind and no expectations.

Chapter Five:
Chakras and Reiki

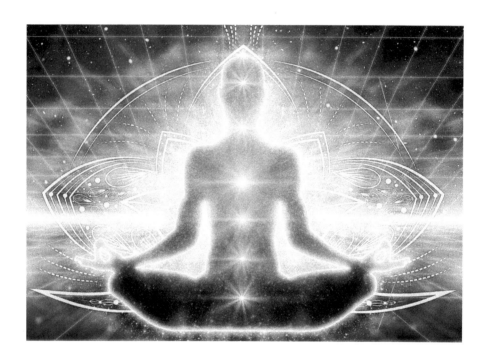

"When you bow, you should just bow. When you sit, you should just sit. When you eat, you should just eat."
- *Shunryu Suzuki*

The chakra system is a huge component of the energetic anatomy in the body. It is the convergence point of the physical body, energetic body, and the emotional body. Chakras are pools of energy, or energetic centers that help the overall energetic flow within the three bodies that make up a person, that make up you.

Since the chakras are primary sources of energy, then they resonate well with Reiki energy. Since an imbalanced chakra can lead to dis-ease and many uncomfortable or debilitating symptoms in the body, and Reiki energy is a healing method that balances energy in the body, then Reiki can help balance the chakras and some root sources of imbalance.

In the human body there are as many as one hundred and fourteen chakras that make up the chakra system. In western traditions and energetic healing, seven chakras known as the 'main chakras' are the focus of energetic healing.

Each of these chakras resonates with a body cavity, emotions, colors, organs, glands, and hormones. These associations are what lead to the manifestation of symptoms when a chakra is imbalanced. Knowing what the chakra associations are can better help you understand what chakras need work or focus.

Since Reiki is intuitive and goes where it is needed, you aren't going to direct the Reiki energy towards a chakra for balancing. However, knowing where the imbalance has occurred can help guide you to the cause of the imbalance. Once it is realigned with Reiki energy, you can work towards making shifts in your life that will prevent the imbalance from coming back.

Most Reiki courses do include information on the chakras. For more in-depth discussion on knowledge on the chakras and chakra healing, be sure to check out another book in this series *Chakras Healing for Beginners.* That book will elaborate on the information in this chapter and give you more knowledge and wisdom to help with balancing our chakras.

When you learn the different static hand positions for a Reiki session, you'll notice that they correspond to the chakras and the body cavities that the seven main chakras align with. This further illustrates how Reiki energy and the chakra system are related. Many Reiki practitioners might even start or end their sessions by placing their hands over the seven main chakras on themselves or on their recipient.

As touched on in a former chapter, the word chakra translates into wheel or disk. Chakras are spinning disks or wheels of energy in the body. They are cone shaped and expand outward, connecting the physical, emotional, and energetic bodies. The chakras have energy that rotates in a clockwise and counterclockwise direction creating a sort of three-dimensional spiral. Chakras are three-dimensional, hence their cone shape.

The seven main chakras run along the spin. The apex, or point of the cone is at the spine and then the chakra cones expand outwards to the front and back of the body. The exceptions to this are the crown chakra which only expands up out of the top of the head and the root chakra which expands down to the feet.

Crown Chakra
The crown chakra is located at the top of the head. It expands up from the cranium and into the universe. The crown chakra connects your personal energy to universal energies and cosmic energies. This is the source of your cosmic consciousness and connects you to divine intelligence and wisdom.

The crown chakra is associated with the color violet or white. It represents bliss, union, and the knowledge that you are one with all else. The crown chakra resonates with peace and cosmic consciousness.

The crown chakra is associated with the mind, brain, nervous system, and the pituitary gland. It is also associated with the hypothalamus. The crown chakra is an element-less chakra. Your crown chakra allows you to access higher states of consciousness and is connected to transcendence of your limitations. Opposites become one in the crown chakra. You can also receive clarity, enlightenment, and wisdom.

When the crown chakra is imbalanced it can present as many different symptoms. It creates feelings of disconnection for the spirit and spiritual energies. A cynical mood about what is sacred can be a result of an imbalanced crown chakra. You may also feel disconnected from your physical body. Other imbalances present as obsessive attachments to spirituality, being close minded, headaches, nightmares, mental illness, and eye problems.

When working with the crown chakra there are some crystals that can enhance the Reiki energy for balancing this chakra. Crystal associations include clear quartz, selenite, diamond, and amethyst.

Third Eye Chakra

Your third eye chakra is between your brows on the front of your body. On the back of your body, the third eye chakra is at the occipital ridge. Your third eye chakra is associated with intuition, awareness, and perception. It provides the energy for spiritual reflection and insights. Through the third eye chakra, you experience clear thought, visions, and independent thought in a strong mind.

The color associated with the third eye chakra is indigo or dark purple. It resonates with the cranial cavity of the body as well as the eyes, nose, and the ears. The third eye chakra resonates with the pituitary gland and helps to regulate hormone production. The third eye chakra is associated with all elements.

This is your intuitive center, your foresight. The third eye chakra is driven by imagination and open mindedness. It can help you see subtle qualities in reality and open you up to different realms and their energies. The third eye chakra closely resonates with dimensions and the spirit worlds. The third eye chakra is also associated with the development of psychic abilities and energetic shifts or movements.

When imbalanced, the third eye chakra can contribute to the feeling of being stuck in a rut. It prevents you from being able to look beyond your own problems. When overactive, the third eye chakra can cause a lack of support from the other chakras. It can create fantasies that are more real and desirable than reality. An imbalanced third eye chakra can also prevent you from being able to see visions of yourself. You might try to reject anything spiritual and have the inability to see the bigger picture. Imbalances can lead to a general lack of clarity, depression, anguish, and mental turmoil.

Crystals that can be used to enhance Reiki energy when working with the third eye chakra include amethyst, fluorite, kyanite, and lapis lazuli.

Throat Chakra

The heart chakra is located at the base of the throat on the front of the body. It is located at the base of the cervical vertebrae on the back of the body, or between two tops of the shoulder blades. Your throat chakra is your center of communication and expression. This is both verbal and non-verbal communication. It is your authentic voice, your truth.

The throat chakra is associated with the thoracic cavity. Its element association is spirit or ether. It resonates with the shoulders, neck, mouth, jaw, tongue, pharynx, larynx, vocal cords, palate, and thyroid gland. The thyroid gland regulates body temperature, growth, and metabolism. The color of the throat chakra is blue.

The throat chakra is all about expressing yourself and expressing your truth. It is closely related to the sacral chakra which is a center of creativity and expression of your identity. The throat chakra is a reference point that connects and aligns with all the body chakras, including main chakras and sub-chakras. In your throat chakra, external and internal communication take place. It also provides you with a connection to etheric realms and helps you to create, bring projects ideas and blueprints into a reality.

When imbalanced, the symptoms of the throat chakra can present as a lack of control with speech. This can be speaking too much or too little, or speech impediments. With an imbalanced throat chakra, you might have difficulty listening to other people or listening to the universe. You may have difficulty keeping secrets, or be very secretive. It can also manifest as compulsive or excessive lying and not being able to keep your word. Other imbalances in the throat chakra include stiff neck, hearing problems, sore throat, and thyroid problems.

Crystals that resonate with the throat chakra include blue lace agate, lapis lazuli, blue jade, blue topaz, and celestite. These crystals can enhance Reiki energy work with the throat chakra.

Heart Chakra

Your heart chakra is located in the center of your sternum in the front of your body and between the center of your shoulder blades, just above the adrenal glands, on the back of your body. It is not directly over the heart organ. The heart chakra is the center of unconditional love and compassion. This is love for yourself, for others, romantic love, familial love, friend love, and an all-encompassing universal love.

Associated with the color green, the heart chakra resonates with the element air. It is closely associated with the diaphragm between the thoracic and abdominal cavities. The heart chakra resonates with the thymus and the lymphatic system. It also correlates to the heart organ, diaphragm, and the lungs. The heart chakra is driven by integration and transformation. It is a bridge between earthly and spiritual aspirations.

Your heart chakra is going to give you deep feelings of connection. It provides harmonious exchanges of energy with everything and everyone around you. It also allows you to see the world and everything in it from a place of love and beauty. A healthy, balanced heart chakra opens you up to giving and receiving love. It is a pure source of unconditional, universal love for everyone and everything, detached from personal biases.

If the heart chakra becomes imbalanced it can lead to difficulty relating to other people and their emotions. Imbalanced heart chakras lead to excessive jealousy, codependency, and being closed down and withdrawn. Other imbalances in the heart chakra can lead to a lack of self-love, lack of self-worth, and a lack of self-confidence. This can lead to fear and self-destructive tendencies.

When working with Reiki and the heart chakra some crystals that can enhance the healing process include rose quartz, green jade, emerald, green calcite, malachite, and rhodonite.

Solar Plexus Chakra

The solar plexus chakra, sometimes called the naval chakra or the third chakra, is located an inch or two above the naval on the front of the body. On the back of the body, the solar plexus chakra is an inch or two above the sacrum in the center of the back. The solar plexus chakra is your will center, your personal power, and your assertiveness. It is the center of yourself, your identity.

From the solar plexus chakra, you get control. You get control over your own path, destiny, and dreams. The solar plexus chakra is associated with the color yellow. Its element is fire, and this is where the term 'fire in your belly' comes from. The solar plexus chakra resonates with the abdominal cavity and the organs that reside there. It is closely related to your stomach, intestines, and the digestive system. It is your center of personal power and will power.

Your inner child resides in your solar plexus chakra. It is also the source of power for your mental abilities and activates your ability to assert yourself into the world. The idea of 'making your mark' in the world comes from your solar plexus chakra. You have a purpose in the world and your solar plexus chakra can help lead you to it. The solar plexus is your personal identity. It is where your assuredness, self-discipline, and independence stems from.

When imbalanced, the solar plexus chakra can lead to symptoms that result in energetic, physical, mental, and emotional illnesses. This includes obsessive compulsive disorders and control issues. An imbalanced solar plexus chakra might present with poor decision-making skills, problems with the immune system and the nervous system as well as low virality.

If you are using Reiki to work with the Solar Plexus chakra, some crystals that can enhance the experience include yellow tourmaline, yellow topaz, pyrite, tiger's eye, and citrine.

Sacral Chakra

Your sacral chakra is located about an inch below your naval on the front of your body and right over your sacrum on the back of your body. The sacral chakra is your pleasure center. It is the source of your passions and desires. This chakra is also associated with sensuality and sexuality. It is sometimes called the sex chakra or the second chakra.

Orange is the color of the sacral chakra and water is its element. The sacral chakra is associated with the abdominopelvic cavity and organs such as the bladder, uterine tract, and other low abdomen organs. It's also associated with the adrenal glands and helps regulate and maintain the immune system. Descriptions for the sacral chakra include flowing and flexible. It is strongly connected to the emotional body which contributes to creativity, pleasure, and sensuality. It is driven by pleasure and the pleasure principle.

The sacral chakra is your emotional center. This is where your sexual orientation and expression of sexual desires stems from. Since it is motivated by pleasure, your sacral chakra is going to encourage you to enjoy life through all of your senses. It wants you to experience the world around you through taste, touch, sound, smell, sight. The sacral chakra is connected to the throat chakra as it is a source of expressing your personal identity. It also supports personal expansion and growth as well as creativity and fantasies.

If the sacral chakra becomes imbalanced, it can present as dependency or codependency on people or substances. You might find yourself being ruled by your emotions or be completely numb and out of touch. Imbalances in the sacral chakra can lead to overindulgences in fantasies. There can be a manifestation of obsessions with sexual intimacy or a lack of interest in sex. You might feel stuck in one mood. Other imbalances in the sacral chakra present as boredom, over-seriousness, resentment, disdain, as well as bladder and uterine disorders.

Crystals that resonate with the sacral chakra and can enhance your Reiki sessions include copper, jasper, carnelian, amber, moonstone, and orange calcite.

Root Chakra

The root chakra is located at the base of the spine. It extends downwards toward the feet. This is your grounding center, your foundation. The root chakra is sometimes called the first chakra. It is linked to your security and survival.

The element of the root chakra is earth and it is a dense chakra. The root chakra is associated with the color red and sometimes black. It resonates with the pelvic cavity and the organs within. The root chakra resonates with the reproductive organs of both men and women, as well as the reproductive hormones. It regulates production as well as sexual development.

Your root chakra is the source of your security. It is the foundation of yourself and for the expansion and growth of life. It is your support system for growth and your anchor for your energies to this world. The root chakra holds your basic needs for survival and is a major contributor to your physicality. It grounds you and holds many aspects of yourself, at least the aspects that make up your foundation.

When imbalanced, the root chakra contributes to excessive negativity. You might become cynical and live inside your illusions. This is often accompanied by feelings of dread and insecurity. You can get trapped in a survival mindset, fight or flight mode. You may become fearful and paranoid. Other symptoms of an imbalanced root chakra include eating disorders, obesity, hemorrhoids, constipation, and any issues with the blood, bones, feet, and legs.

If you are using Reiki energy to work with the root chakra, some crystals that resonate with the root chakra include smoky quartz, garnet, ruby, black tourmaline, obsidian, jet, and onyx.

Chapter Six:
Reiki Healing and Self-Healing

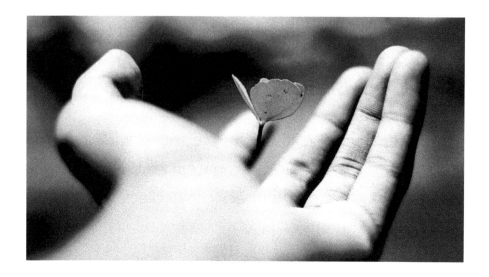

"You can't stop the waves, but you can learn to surf."
- Jon Kabat-Zinn

Reiki energy healing is a profoundly powerful tool when healing yourself and also when healing others. It might seem easier to seek out a Reiki practitioner, however, there are different benefits to performing Reiki sessions on yourself.

That being said, there are also benefits to receiving Reiki sessions from practitioners as well. Depending on what your goals are, what your intentions are, and what you have been feeling or going through, is going to be a factor when looking at what method is going to work best for you.

When all said and done, generally utilizing a combination of the ways you can receive and apply Reiki is going to be of the greatest benefit. Of course, the best and most powerful healing comes from within, so implementing daily self-treatment Reiki sessions is always going to be encouraged and recommended.

Depending on where you live, you might find it difficult to find a Reiki practitioner. That isn't necessarily a bad thing. Many Reiki practitioners offer distance and online services and sessions. A distance Reiki session is just as powerful as an in-person session and can yield the same results. Some people find distance sessions to be preferred as they tend to have a little more flexibility around busy or strict schedules.

There are some basic and overall benefits of Reiki healing. The most profound and common benefits that you can receive from Reiki treatments include:

- Promoting harmony and balance
- Promotes deep relaxation, allowing the body to release stress and tension
- Aligns energy imbalances and promotes a balance between body, mind, and spirit
- Cleanses the body and organs of toxins and boosts the immune system
- Clears the mind and improves focus
- Grounds and centers
- Assists with sleep
- Improves the body's ability to heal itself
- Relieves pain and supports healing of the physical body
- Guides in spiritual growth and emotional cleansing
- Compliments medical treatments and therapies for other conditions

Along with well documented benefits of Reiki energy healing, there are also some disease and conditions that have been known to be benefited when treated with Reiki alongside their medical treatments.

Some common medical diagnoses that have shown improvement or been benefited with Reiki include:

- Cancer
- Heart Disease
- Anxiety
- Depression
- Chronic Pain
- Infertility
- Neurodegenerative Diseases
- Autism
- Crohn's Disease
- Fatigue Syndromes

The uses for Reiki healing are innumerable. Even when just seeking to improve your awareness, personal power, and raising your energetic vibration, Reiki becomes such an asset in every day life. There are thousands of reasons to use Reiki energy to heal yourself and very few reasons not to.

The rest of this chapter is going to take a look at different ways Reiki energy can be used for healing, their differences, and their potential benefits. Overtime, you will learn to follow your intuition and the wisdom of Reiki to follow the path that is best for you. Having the correct knowledge and information on different types of Reiki healing sessions is going to help you on that path.

Self- Treatment Sessions

A self-treatment session with Reiki energy can be performed after you receive your Reiki Level I attunement ceremony. In a later chapter, the hand positions for a self-treatment session will be covered, but you can always adapt and change the hand positions to whatever feels right or comfortable.

When performing a Reiki self-treatment, you'll want to make sure that you are in a quiet, relaxed space where you can be undisturbed for around forty-five minutes. This is one benefit to self-treatment sessions, you have more control over how long the session will last. You will also be able to fit them in on your own schedule rather than trying to coordinate with a practitioner and their schedule.

While you can be sitting up or lying down for a Reiki self-treatment, if you are prone to falling asleep when lying down and relaxing, you might want to perform self-treatments while sitting up.

One of the beauties of Reiki energy is that when you perform a session on yourself, or even on someone else, you are drawing Reiki energy from the universe. You are not expending any of your personal energy, so after a session you should not feel physically depleted or exhausted. If you were tired before performing a self-treatment session, you may in fact feel more awake and alert when the session is complete.

That is another benefit of self-treatment sessions, if you need a boost after work to get through your evening activities, doing a self-treatment session can provide you with that energetic pick-me up you might need.

As has been touched on a few times, the best healing comes from within. This means that you are the most instrumental source of your own healing. Self-treatment sessions give you the power to pursue that internal healing process. Even when you get Reiki healing sessions from another practitioner, you are still going to have to look within for the sources of imbalances and for the proper way to shift your energy and prevent future imbalances.

When performing self-treatment sessions with Reiki your intuition is going to be much more aligned with what is happening inside your own body. Therefore, you can get to the root of your imbalance faster and discover what will work for you in fixing it.

The body has such an amazing ability to heal itself. Unfortunately, modern societies impose limitations, jobs, and other restrictions that tend to work against the body's natural ability to heal itself. By aligning your personal energy flow and changing your energetic vibration, you are giving your body the means to heal itself. This healing happens on a physical, emotional, and spiritual level.

Reiki is a holistic healing energy. That means it heals all, it heals and balances on all levels of all the components of the body. Treating yourself with Reiki energy every day is going to keep your body in that alignment, so that you can focus more on your desires and goals in life and not sicken yourself with worry, stress, or be bogged down by physical pain.

Self-treatment sessions are great because of the flexibility in time and schedule that they offer you. Self-treatment sessions give you more control over hand positions and what is done in a session, or what Reiki symbols are used, if you've been attuned to Reiki symbols. Self-treatment sessions allow you to heal yourself from within, which is the most profound way to heal yourself.

Healing Crisis

Sometimes when going through the process of self-healing and shifting your own vibration, you can encounter what is called a Healing Crisis.

A healing crisis occurs when you begin a new course of study, or treatment, or pursue a new field of education, such as Reiki, and things don't seem to go as 'planned.'

An example could be that you experience chronic inflammation. This inflammation starts due to a single stressor to the body which results in a defensive response i.e. inflammation. This stressor can be physical, emotional, external, or internal.

If the stressor is not identified and you continue to use the substance, practice the action, or follow the belief that triggered the inflammation, then the problem is just going to get worse. Your defense reaction will happen again and again, building on that inflammation until it becomes chronic.

Let's say that before you were dealing with the inflammation your body, mind, and spirit were operating at a level of 7 or 8 on a scale of 1 to 10, on most days. Now that the inflammation has become chronic, perhaps you are functioning more at a 4 or a 5 on a scale of 1 to 10 every day. You begin to adjust and learn to live with that chronic condition because it just becomes a part of you.

Suddenly, change can take place. It has been recommended that you try a new vitamin, that you talk to a new therapist, or that you look into a new course of study. You decide to give it a go. Initially, you might not feel any change and you could assume that it just didn't work. In some cases, you might find that you feel worse and you attribute the worsening feelings to the new method you tried.

This type of healing crisis is a common problem. What happens is, as the body, mind, and spirit are exploring something new or learning something new, it causes you to take a step back. The intention of the step back is to adjust your perception or perspective. This can sometimes happen when going through Reiki sessions and treatments.

It is important to remember that Reiki is not a heal all, nor it is an instant cure or fix. Reiki energy takes time to work. Additionally, it takes time to understand what needs to be shifted and changed to work towards a healthier lifestyle. Often times, if something doesn't work right away, people give up on it. That is why Reiki self-treatment sessions become so important!

Through treating yourself you can help your mind shift perspectives so that you truly get what you need from the path you are on. Self-treatments on a daily basis can result in more noticeable changes in your day to day life. This is why it is recommended that you document shifts and changes, no matter how subtle.

When you embark on a journey to heal yourself and strive towards a successful, fulfilled existence, a lot can happen. Emotions and traumas can be released, the work can seem slow and fruitless, but truly making a change in yourself isn't going to be easy or quick.

Some things to remember if you feel that you are experiencing a healing crisis are to:

- Be Gentle with Yourself
- Meditate
- Hydrate
- Breathe
- Surrender
- Perform Self-Treatments

Receiving Reiki from another Practitioner

There are many reasons to receive a Reiki session from an experienced practitioner. One of the major reasons to see a practitioner is because you feel blocked. This doesn't mean that you have an energy block, it means that you physically feel blocked in whatever you are experiencing and you are completely unable to help yourself.

Even with all the tools of Reiki self-treatments, crystal healing, and healing the chakras, you might encounter some traumas that cannot be resolved without a little help. If this happens, seeing a Reiki practitioner for sessions is a great way to help you move past that block enough so that you can start healing yourself. In this case, having a Reiki practitioner work on you is going to jump start your ability to work on yourself.

You may need to go for several sessions, or find that you want to continue seeing your Reiki practitioner as you work on yourself as well.

Other reasons to see another Reiki practitioner can be about experience and technique. You can learn a lot about Reiki by receiving sessions from another practitioner. You can learn new techniques and also discover new methods of applying Reiki. Everyone has differing experience levels and a lot of Reiki practitioners learn multiple energetic disciplines that you might find interesting.

Another reason to have a Reiki practitioner is for a sense of community. There are a lot of Reiki communities in local settings now. Joining a Reiki community is a great way to meet like minded people, share techniques and knowledge, and some Reiki communities trade free sessions when they meet.

This is just the beginning, you are going to keep learning and growing, so having other Reiki practitioners that can offer guidance and wisdom is such an asset.

Even if you become a Reiki Master, it is still recommended that you get Reiki sessions from other Reiki practitioners. The frequency of this is going to be a personal choice, however you shouldn't replace your self-treatment sessions with sessions from another practitioner.

It isn't uncommon for practitioners to have multiple other practitioners that they see for sessions. If you recall, after the 1980s, it was encouraged for Reiki students to study under different masters and receive Reiki sessions from different practitioners. Not only you can learn from them, but they can learn from you as well. It becomes an exchange of knowledge and growth for the both of you.

When looking for Reiki practitioners in your area, you'll want to find ones that you feel a connection to, that you resonate with. You might decide that you want to have some in-person practitioners, but then also have a Reiki practitioner that performs distance healing sessions. This continues to expand your Reiki network and your healing opportunities. Sometimes your intuition will guide you to a practitioner for a specific reason, but lead you to a different practitioner for another reason.

Many Reiki practitioners refine themselves to a specialty or a niche. For example, some practitioners will work only with clients who experience chronic pain. Others will work with clients specifically on healing past life and generational traumas. Other practitioners might focus on clients with mental illness such as depression or anxiety disorders.

There are many different reasons to get a healing session from someone else, and one of the most important reasons is because it feels good and is very beneficial.

Performing Reiki Sessions on Other People
When you perform a Reiki session on someone else, two things happen. The first is that you provide a widely beneficial healing service to a recipient who is in need. The second thing that happens is when you channel the

Reiki energy through yourself you retain Reiki benefits for yourself, even if your focus is on your client. Definitely a win-win situation.

When performing Reiki on others, it is important to get their permission. That may sound obvious, but if you get attuned to Reiki Level II and have the ability to perform distance sessions, you won't need a client on your table to provide healing services. That being said, you always want permission from a recipient before performing a session. Without permission, you could unintentionally push someone into processing emotions they aren't ready to process which can have negative results.

Performing Reiki sessions on someone else has benefits for you that go beyond just channeling Reiki energy through yourself. Since Reiki is channeled energy through you, performing Reiki sessions on others won't drain you of energy. You shouldn't be putting your personal energy into a Reiki session, it should all come from the channeling of universal energy. When you act as the conduit for Reiki energy, you are a one-way conduit. That means as energy shifts and releases from your client, it can't travel back through the conduit into your body. Many other energy healing methods don't have that built in safety feature, so practitioners can inadvertently pickup energies that are released from the recipients. Reiki has not such risk.

Another benefit to performing Reiki sessions on other people is in the learning. By working on others, your intuition can lead you to different hand positions and techniques that you might not discover while working on yourself only. Additionally, since clients and recipients will have different reasons for healing than you, your knowledge and understanding of energy and root causes of imbalances is going to expand and grow.

Having that wisdom will only help you as you progress on your own healing path. The point of self-healing isn't just to improve your physical, emotional, and spiritual health, but to allow you to grow and change with the knowledge and wisdom that you gain. Performing Reiki sessions on other people gives you the opportunity for literal hands on learning experiences.

Sometimes it takes working on another person to experience visions and sensations related to energetic shifts in the body. While working on yourself you can often feel the shifts occurring in your body, if you feel them in someone else, it takes your understanding of Reiki to a much deeper level.

Most practitioners who decide to provide Reiki healing services professionally to clients will rise up to at least Reiki Level II. It isn't necessary; however, it is recommended. If you don't want to offer professional services, you can still use the knowledge from Reiki Level I to offer complimentary healing services to friends and family or in a Reiki community.

Chapter Seven:
Reiki Healing Techniques

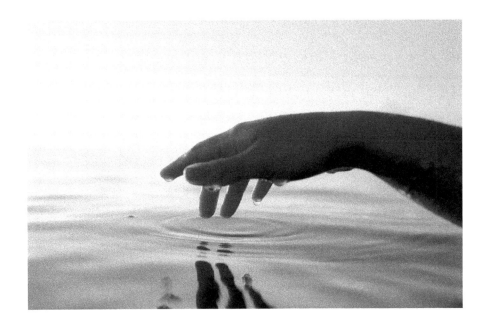

"Do every act of your life as if it were the very last act of your life."
- *Marcus Aurelius*

When it comes to performing Reiki sessions on yourself and on others there are many different methods and techniques that can be applied. There are a basic set of hand positions that are commonly utilized for beginners. However, as you continue to practice you might find hand positions that resonate with you better or that you find more comfortable.

The way you start and end your session is going to vary as well. You'll find your own routine and methods for performing Reiki sessions. Having a starting point is going to be beneficial in the early stages of your learning and practicing Reiki.

Self-Reiki Treatments

Before you perform a Reiki treatment session on yourself, you are going to want to establish a space for your self-treatment. There are no right or wrong ways to set up your self-treatment space. Some people will perform Reiki sessions on themselves in the same place where they meditate. Other people might have a designated space for Reiki sessions only.

You'll want to make sure that you have a quiet, undisturbed space where you can be alone for about forty-five minutes. You'll want the environment to be relaxing. If that means including calm music, candles, incense, dim lighting, or a nice warm blanket, make the space yours, however you define relaxing.

Self-treatments can be performed while sitting up or while lying down. If you think you might fall asleep while lying down, perform them sitting up. If you do fall asleep during a self-treatment session, the next time that you perform a session, pickup where you last remember leaving off on the session you fell asleep in.

Before starting a self-treatment, wash your hands in cold water to help clear them as a channel for Reiki energy. Once you are comfortable in your space, you'll want to take several deep breaths. As you breathe deeply, let go of any intentions or expectations for the Reiki session. Simply ask that Reiki energy flow through you and then begin your hand positions. You'll want to start at your head and then work your way down the body.

The following picture is a basic outline of what the hand positions for a self-Reiki treatment can look like. You can adapt of change the hand positions as you feel called to.

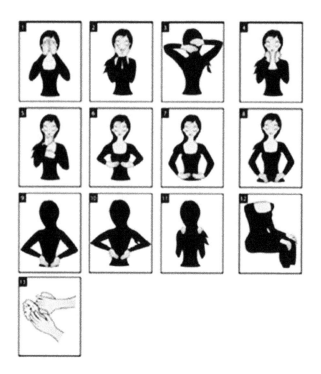

During a self-Reiki treatment, you'll want to hold each position for between three and five minutes. Let your intuition guide you on how long to hold each position. You might find that some feel like they should be held longer while others don't. The hand positions that feel like they should be held longer can change over time as well.

Once you work through all the Reiki hand positions, you'll want to take a few more deep breaths. Before ending the session give thanks to the Reiki energy and then intend that the session is over. You might want to place your palms or forehead on the floor to help ground yourself after a session. You can also wash your hands in cold water after a session to help clear and ground you as well.

At the beginning or end of every self-treatment session, some practitioners like to place their hands over each of the seven main chakras. This just helps the mind consciously activate these chakras.

When performing Reiki on yourself, you might want to begin and/or end your session with a Gassho mediation for fifteen or so minutes. This can really help you open up to Reiki and help you focus on balance and gratitude for the duration of the session.

You could begin each Reiki session with Reiji-Ho as well to help you connect deeper with Reiki and to enhance the session. Chiyro can also be a wonderful addition to any self-Reiki treatment session.

There are other additives that can boost a self-treatment session to help you maximize your healing. One common and fairly easy to incorporate additive is in using crystals in your Reiki sessions. Whether you place a crystal directly on your body, use a crystal grid, or hold a crystal in your hand for a treatment session, the energy of the crystal will be included in the Reiki session.

For more information on crystal properties and how to use them with Reiki read about them in the book *Crystals Healing for Beginners*. Crystals do have individual properties, so if you'd like to use them in your Reiki sessions, you'll want to make sure you are using crystals with corresponding properties.

Getting into a routine with how you start and end your self-Reiki treatment sessions is going to help you stick to a daily routine with your sessions. As always, let your intuition guide you through the sessions. You may feel the desire or need to include Gassho in one session and then not the next. Listen to that intuitive voice because the body knows what it needs, regardless of how much the conscious mind tries to convince it that it doesn't.

When using Reiki on yourself, you can place your hands directly on your body, or you can hold your hands a few inches away from the body. Both are effective methods of performing a session. If you are attuned to Reiki Level

II, you might be called to include Reiki power symbols in a self-treatment session.

Reiki power symbols can be visualized and beamed into a specific area. Power symbols can be drawn directly over a part of the body. Intoning a power symbol three time is how you can activate it for your Reiki session. Intoning can be verbal or mental.

Aromatherapy is another complimenting additive when it comes to self-Reiki sessions. You can use essential oils in a diffuser, scented incense, or dilute essential oils in a carrier oil and place them directly on your skin. Not only do essential oils and herbal incense smell lovely, aromatherapy is a great way to connect with natural plant energies and their healing properties.

If you don't want to use addition tools like crystals and essential oils, there are other ways to enhance a session that don't require any tools at all. During a self-Reiki session, using affirmations and manifestations can really bring clarity and meaning to the sessions. Affirming that you receive the balance you need from a self-treatment session is going to super-charge your Reiki session.

Manifesting balanced chakras during a Reiki session just adds to the healing power.

After performing a self-treatment, take some time to write down everything you experienced, felt, saw, or any other sensations you had during the session. Try keeping a journal or notebook nearby where you perform sessions on yourself for easy access. This is going to be important, especially when you first start performing session on yourself.

Sometimes, you might find that you need a quick Reiki session, but you aren't in your treatment space. Maybe you are still at work, or driving down the road, or out with friends. A situation might arise where you get a headache or feel tired and sluggish, or your foot cramps up. Maybe it is during your menstruation cycle and you are experiencing severe pain.

Performing a quick five to ten-minute Reiki session on yourself is going to help you get over that obstacle. To start the session, you'll want to ask for Reiki energy to start flowing through you. Then place your hands where you think they are most needed. For a headache, maybe you'll place them on either side of your head, for menstrual cramps, maybe you'll rest your hands on your lower abdomen. Then allow the Reiki to flow for five to ten minutes before giving thanks to Reiki energy and ending the session.

These quick sessions during your day shouldn't become a substitute for full self-Reiki treatment sessions. However, they can provide quick relief or a small boost during your day.

Sometimes you might see or feel something that doesn't make sense during the session, but after writing it down and analyzing the personal symbolism, you'll understand what it means and how to use it. Other times, having a written progression of your personal progress is going to be a validating account of the shifts and changes that that are being made.

Reiki is a skill. The more you practice, the more you learn and the more comfortable it becomes.

Reiki Treatments for Others

Even if you don't intend to perform Reiki sessions on others in a professional setting, you should still have an understanding on the best way to perform sessions on others, or the different ways you can perform sessions on other people. This will give you insight into whether or not you really want to provide Reiki sessions for others, or maybe help guide you in what level of Reiki you want to study to.

Healing Space

If you are planning on performing Reiki healing sessions for people in a professional setting, it is important to have a healing space. This space should be exclusively for healing clients. If you are making a career out of it, renting an office space where you can set up is ideal. If you have the space in your home, you can also designate an area for Reiki sessions in your home.

You'll want a treatment table, such as a massage table. Massage tables are designed for comfort and come with a face cradle so you can turn your clients over and work on their backs allowing them to have a comfortable place to rest their head and faces.

The space itself should be clean and well kept. You'll want to decorate it in a way that is relaxing and inviting. Bubblegum pink walls probably aren't the most relaxing, but a nice soothing beige or white speaks more to a relaxing environment for the mind. If the space has windows, having heavy curtains to block out sun is important. Your recipient is going to by lying on a table and they don't want to have sun shining into their eyes.

You'll want sheets and a blanket for your treatment table as some people will get cold or feel more comfortable with the pressure of sheets and blankets on top of them. When it comes to sheets, solid colors tend to be the best. Dinosaur or Captain America sheets might not send the most professional, relaxing intention in that space.

Other decorations might include pictures and wall hangings, flowers, electric candles, and crystals. You'll want the space to reflect your own energy, but also to provide a safe, relaxing, calm, and secure environment.

In your healing space, it is a good idea to have a couple chairs. One reason is that when you first meet your clients, you'll probably want to talk to them and get to know them as well as their reasons for coming to see you for Reiki. Having a comfortable chair for them to sit in is going to be more inviting. Having a chair for yourself so you aren't standing over them is also another inviting gesture.

While diffusing essential oils and burning incense or smudge sticks can be very relaxing, be aware that some people are sensitive to strong scents or have allergies.

This extends to personal hygiene as well. When performing a session on yourself, you are going to be up close and personal to your client. You'll want to avoid strong scented perfumes and deodorant, as well as keeping your teeth brushed and making sure your nails are clipped and filed.

Another important consideration when it comes to your Reiki practice space is that you'll want a method of clearing the space before each session, or at least at the beginning of the day and end of the day. Energy that is released can get hung up in corners or on objects in your healing space. Regular clearing will keep the space positive and healthy for yourself and your clients.

Performing A Healing Session for Others
Before you perform an in-person Reiki session on someone else, you'll want a basic understanding of why they have come to you for healing services and what their knowledge of Reiki is. If they don't know about Reiki, be

prepared to answer question and offer a little information on the history and concepts of Reiki.

Having a professional attitude and being open to answering their questions will help them relax and help you connect to them. Clients like practitioners who are knowledgeable enough to answer their queries.

A Reiki session can be performed with your client completely clothed. You may want to establish prior to starting the session whether they are comfortable with you touching with or if they would rather have you hold your hands above their body for the session. You'll want to strive towards your client's comfort and start building a trust bond with them.

Before you touch your client or perform Reiki on them, wash your hands with soap in cold water. This is to help clear your hands for the Reiki energy, but also for hygiene purposes. Anytime you are touching someone, you should be washing your hands before and after.

Start your Reiki session by letting go of intentions and expectations for the session. Ask that Reiki energy flow through you. This is the point of the session where you can implement the Reiji-Ho or Chiyro pillar when working with a client. Then you can begin the hand positions on your client. The below picture is an outline of the basic hand positions to use when performing a Reiki treatment on someone else.

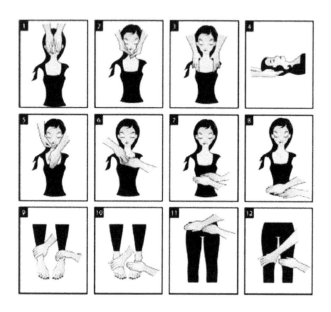

You'll want to hold each position for three to five minutes, or as long as your intuition calls. When moving from one position to another, lift your hands and then place them down gently in the next position. Sliding your hands from one position to another can be somewhat unsettling for a client.

Starting from the head, you'll work your way down the body and end near the feet. You can also flip your client onto their stomach and use hand positions on their back if you are called to do so. There are a few positions on the body that you are going to want to take your hands off your client, if they are allowing you to touch them. Holding your hands over the pubic bone and over the coccyx are powerful positions, but they are close to the genitalia and right above the gluteus muscles so you don't want to be touching them directly.

When touching someone for healing, be gentle. Don't press your hands down firmly or drop them down onto parts of their body. Also practice Mindful Touch. What this means is that while you are working on a client, be focused on your client. Don't be thinking about what you're making for dinner or when the dog was last taken for a walk. Be mindful that you are working on another human and your intention and focus should be on them.

Recipients can feel if you aren't focused on a session, and it can become quite an unpleasant and unsatisfactory experience. Mindful touch is important to the benefit of a Reiki session as well as creating a trust bond with your clients.

When you have completed your hand positions, you might want to end the session by touching each of your client's chakras. You'll also want to close your client to the energetic flow. You can do this by fluffing their aura, or by placing the pointer and middle fingers of each hand above the third eye and sacral chakras and then lifting up away from their body.

Once your client is closed, you'll want to give thanks to Reiki energy and your client. You'll want to let them know the session is over and invite them to take their time getting up. In some cases, you might need to help your client sit or stand up after a session.

You'll want to wash your hands with soap and cold water again to ground and clear yourself. It is a good practice to offer your clients a glass of water after a session. You'll also want to leave time to discuss the session with them and discuss a treatment plan going forward.

Just like with self-treatment sessions, you can include crystals and aromatherapy into Reiki sessions. However, these are tools that you want to discuss using with your clients first as not everyone is open to crystals and aromatherapy.

Including affirmations and manifestations in a Reiki session performed on someone are both acceptable enhancements. You might include Chiyro at the beginning or end of your Reiki session as an added technique for amplifying and maximizing the healing that your client receives.

Group Sessions
Group sessions are when multiple practitioners perform a single session on one client. You may not get the change to perform a group session, but if you join a Reiki community, then the chances are probably higher.

Before performing a group session you'll want to establish with the other practitioners how you are going to transition through the hand positions, so that the session flows smoothly and people aren't tripping over each other.

Group sessions are powerful and expose one client to many different energetic frequencies. If you do get the chance to participate in a group session, take it. It is a unique Reiki experience.

Distance Reiki Sessions

Once you are attuned to Reiki Level II and the Reiki power symbols, you can perform distance Reiki sessions. Reiki can be sent through time and space, and when activated by the proper distance Reiki symbol, you can perform complete sessions on clients.

There are a few different methods for performing a Reiki distance session. One way is to have a doll or a stuffed animal that represents your client. Prior to performing the session, you'll want to set the intention that the surrogate is going to represent your client. Stating their name helps.

Then you will go through the motions and hand positions of a regular session but performing it on your surrogate doll or stuffed animal.

Another distance Reiki session method is to use your own body to represent your client. You'll want to set the intention at the beginning of the session that your body is representing your client. Once the intention is set, you can begin performing the session with the self-Reiki treatment hand positions.

The third option for Reiki distance sessions is to have a picture of your client and intend that the picture is going to represent their body. Then go through the hand positions of a Reiki session.

As with any Reiki session, you'll want to wash your hands in cold water before and after the session. Distance sessions can also include crystals, aromatherapy, affirmations, manifestations, and the incorporation of Reiji-Ho and Chiyro. Distance sessions are just as powerful and adaptable as in person sessions.

Reiki and Past Life Healing

Since Reiki can be sent through time and space, it can also be used to heal past life traumas. Some people carry past life traumas into their current life cycle. When this happens, they may not be able to discover the source of their imbalances. With the Reiki distance symbol, you can send Reiki back through their past lives and use your intuition to guide you.

This can be very deep work and should only be done with clients that are ready and serious about the healing. Past life work can bring up a lot of emotions, memories, and experiences that don't always make sense. It can be profoundly beneficial, but it can also be heavy. If you want to use Reiki to heal past lives, study the concept of past lives and methods for healing them along with your Reiki studies.

Chapter Eight:
Physical Healing

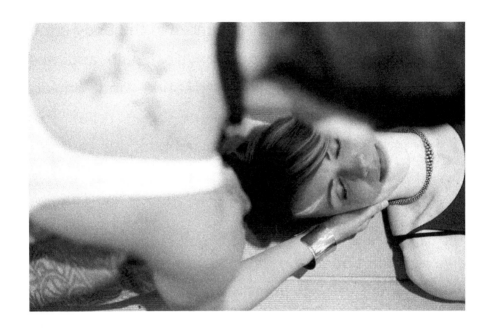

"Treat everyone you meet as if they were you."
- Doug Dillon

Reiki is a holistic healing practice. That means it can heal the physical body, emotional/mental body, and the spiritual body. When it comes to physical healing, it is easy to think that the body need medicine or massage or physical manipulation to heal physical pain or physical diseases.

This isn't always the case. Imbalances in the body create dis-ease, which then leads to physical pain and even illness and disease. While medication and physical manipulation of the body might offer relief from symptoms, healing has to go straight to the source in order for the healing to truly be effective.

Reiki is not a miracle cure. It is not a heal all method. However, the benefits that Reiki offers sometimes give the body what it needs in order to find its balance, relief, and healing. There are no guarantees, but Reiki is powerful and can accomplish great things in the body.

That being said, Reiki is a wonderful compliment to medical treatments as it can help reduce side effects from medications and therapies, as well as quicken the recovery process. In the cases of terminal illness, Reiki can become a huge asset in easing pain, providing comfort, and aiding in the mental and emotional implications that arise.

For more serious diseases, treatment can be hard and long and painful. Reiki may not be able to completely cure these diseases, but providing comfort and relieving the emotional, physical, and mental stresses makes a drastic difference for the patient.

This is becoming so apparent that many nurses are taking Reiki courses and getting attuned to Reiki so that they can perform it on their patients in hospitals.

Some diseases and physical ailments that can benefit from Reiki include:

- Cancer
- Heart Disease
- Chronic Pain
- Infertility
- Neurodegenerative Diseases
- Crohn's Disease
- Fibromyalgia
- Surgical Recovery

Cancer

Most people know someone who has been affected by cancer. Whether they've lost someone to cancer, know someone who has survived or is in remission, or have experienced cancer themselves. There are so many kinds of cancers and they are aggressive, usually fast, and can result in a lot of physical and emotional symptoms.

The treatments for cancer are hard. They can sometimes result in more horrible side effects than the disease itself.

Patients who are going through cancer treatments can lose their appetite, be in constant pain, feel depressed, anxious, scared, and sometimes be completely alone.

When the body is fighting for survival or trying to heal itself, it is so important to be in a healthy state of mind with emotions and be in a spiritually healthy place. The body does have an incredible power to heal itself, but if there are imbalances and the emotions and spirit begin to experience symptoms then the body has to work three times as hard and it essentially runs out of gas.

When being treated for cancer, the body can be in so much pain that getting a light, relaxing massage is too much.

Since Reiki can be performed with holding then hands over the body, it offers a pleasant, non-invasive alternative to therapies that require touch.

There are many documented cases where people who were diagnosed with cancer chose to stick to alternative therapies. When being treated with Reiki there are many cases in which patients went into remission with just the healing power of Reiki. This doesn't happen in every case, and Reiki isn't a miracle cure, however, it has been known to happen. Either that or a cancerous tumor might show significant slowing in growth or even reduction in size as a result of Reiki sessions.

More importantly, Reiki can relieve the side effects of cancer treatments like radiation and chemotherapy. Reiki can help stimulate the digestive system and appetite, curb nausea and headaches, and release negative emotions of depression, fear, and anxiety.

Sometimes the body and mind benefit more from a relief of the symptoms than a flat-out cure to an underlying disease.

Some cancer patients went into remission with Reiki sessions and continue to get Reiki as a preventative measure and have been living with no additional signs of cancer for years.

In other situations, the toll of depression on the body from going through cancer treatments is so debilitating that the person may start to deteriorate faster and get sick faster. Relieving the depression with Reiki then allows the body to benefit from the cancer treatments.

It can also be beneficial to the family members of cancer patients who are trying to stay brave and strong, but feel depressed and overwhelmed. Reiki sessions can help relieve their emotional symptoms as they are watching a loved one suffers. You can see there are multiple ways that Reiki can be beneficial to cancer patients and their families.

Heart Disease

When it comes to heart disease, there are several underlying causes. These include blood pressure, cholesterol, lifestyle, and genetics. Reiki can't heal genetics, unfortunately. However, Reiki is known to lower blood pressure and lower cholesterol which contribute to and promote heart health.

Many heart diseases are a result of long-term imbalances in the body or long-term unhealthy habits. While it is best to focus on changing your lifestyle to prevent complications down the road, like sticking to a healthier diet, not smoking, and reducing stress when possible, Reiki is another good preventative.

Because Reiki corrects imbalances in the body, it can become a preventative treatment for diseases and ailments that take a long time to build up. Of course, as with any preventative, adjusting your own habits and lifestyle is going to be beneficial as well. Reiki can start and help maintain the process while you also create shifts in your own life.

Reiki can be used in conjunction with blood pressure and cholesterol medications. Since it can lower blood pressure and cholesterol, getting tested regularly while getting Reiki treatments is recommended so the dosages of medication can be adjusted as needed.

Chronic Pain

Chronic pain refers to any instance of constant physical pain that the body experiences. Chronic pain can be in any part of the body and can manifest in many ways. It might be a stabbing pain, burning pain, or a tingling, needle like pain. Anyone who suffers from chronic pain knows how debilitating it can be.

Furthermore, the western medical system isn't really designed to help people with chronic pain that doesn't fall into a predetermined category. What this means is that if there is no 'obvious' source of pain, doctors have a hard time diagnosing it.

People who suffer from chronic pain might have had an accident or injury that triggered the pain, or might feel it because of the job they work. There are so many causes of chronic pain and so few resolutions if it isn't a cookie cutter, common problem.

Unfortunately, this means that many people who suffer from chronic pain end up on long-term regimens of pain killers and muscle relaxants. These medications can in turn have side effects that can become dangerous and debilitating.

These experiences with medication and no diagnosis can become frustrating and discouraging leading to emotional and mental symptoms as well.

Fortunately, Reiki energy healing, doesn't need a diagnosis or a known cause to help relieve chronic pain. With static hand positions, or performing Reiki hands off, you have the ability to provide clients or yourself with pain relief without aggravating it by moving the body or even touching the body.

Because Reiki is intuitive and corrects the imbalances in the body, it goes exactly where it is needed. In the case of chronic pain, if there was no obvious trigger, like a physical trauma or accident, sometimes it is a result of an imbalance somewhere else.

For example, there have been cases of clients seeking massage therapy for pain in their feet. The pain is so bad they can barely walk. Through the course of treatments, and in working backwards from where the pain is felt, the source of the pain is traced back to a surgical scar on the low back from fourteen years earlier.

Situations like this are common. Surgeries can be traumatic to the body and as a defense mechanism, muscles and connective tissues jam up. After the surgery heals, those tissues and muscles stay condensed. Over time, that defense reaction spreads down the legs and continues to jam up muscle and connective tissue until it manifests as severe pain in the feet.

With Reiki and chronic pain, it is not uncommon to have to work backwards from where the pain manifests to where the pain originates. Doctors don't always have the insight beyond the scope of their specialty to find the true source of chronic pain.

Many people who have suffered from chronic pain for years will start getting Reiki sessions and suddenly not have to take pain killers any more, or get to lower the dose, or even go from heavy prescriptions to just basic Ibuprofen.

Infertility

Infertility is another highly emotional condition that people can encounter. Women wanting to have children but being unable to do so is such an emotional experience that it can lead to depression, anxiety, reclusively, and a complete lack of self-worth and self-appreciation.

There are many causes for infertility. Sometimes it is something to do with the woman's body and sometimes it has to do with the man's body. Science can help determine if sperm count is low or if there is a potential problem with the uterus or ovaries. Unfortunately, this doesn't always make the situation better or less emotionally painful.

Any woman that has ever experienced infertility yet who wants to be pregnant knows just how horrible it is to get their period every month, a regular reminder that they aren't pregnant. This kind of physical condition has severe emotional and spiritual implications as well.

Reiki energy can vastly improve the emotional mindset and wellbeing of women and men who are struggling with infertility. Just like with cancer, when that emotional and spiritual energy comes back into alignment, the body can focus on healing itself.

More than that, Reiki can help heal imbalances in both men and women so help the production and secretion of fertility hormones and improve their chances of getting pregnant.

There are many accounts of women who had tried everything to get pregnant and were going through fertility treatments with no luck. After receiving Reiki healing sessions, they would suddenly get a viable embryo for the first time in years! It sounds almost like magic, but the truth is, the body is capable of healing itself in many instances. Reiki just points the way.

As with cancer, Reiki isn't a miracle cure for infertility and sometimes can only treat the emotional and spiritual symptoms rather than the core cause, but never underestimate the difference a positive mindset can make.

Neurodegenerative Disease
Dementia, Parkinson's Disease, and Alzheimer's Disease are some of the most well-known neurodegenerative diseases. There are no cures to these diseases, only treatments.

A neurodegenerative disease occurs in the brain when the brain's ability to communicate with parts of the body begins to deteriorate. As with dementia and Alzheimer's disease, the memory is severely impacted. People lose entire chunks of their lives and their pasts. They can forget family members, spouses, and lifelong friends. More than that they could lose the ability to tie their own shoes because the memory just doesn't exist in their mind anymore.

For neurodegenerative diseases like Parkinson's disease, the brain is no longer capable of communicating with the body and patients begin to lose the function of their body and motor skills.

It is incredibly difficult to watch someone suffer from a neurodegenerative disease and even more difficult to go through it.

Reiki energy healing can actually help slow the degeneration of the neurons and help relieve the physical symptoms of such diseases. There is still a lot to be learned about Reiki and neurodegenerative diseases, but there are documented cases in with Reiki helped to slow the progression of symptoms.

More than that, Reiki provides pain relief for the neurodegenerative diseases that do result in physical pain. Additionally, family members watching someone suffer a neurodegenerative disease can become frustrated, upset, sad, scared, and depressed.

As with cancer, Reiki can benefit those who are watching a loved one suffer from a neurodegenerative disease by relieving their own emotional symptoms. Some neurodegenerative diseases are genetic, so having a parent or family member be diagnosed with one can create a sense of worry and dread in younger members of the family who think that is what they have to look forward to. Reiki can help release that worry and help improve mindfulness about living in the moment and not worrying about what can't be controlled.

Crohn's Disease

Crohn's Disease is an autoimmune, inflammatory disease of the digestive tract. It most commonly effects the intestines and bowels, yet it can also create a sensitivity in the stomach and every other parts of the digestive system.

An autoimmune disease is the result of the body thinking that something that should be there shouldn't be. When this happens, the immune system starts to attack the body and try to fight off whatever is causing the perceived problem. As a result, many other debilitating and problematic symptoms occur.

In the case of Crohn's disease, the digestive trace becomes incredibly overactive and starts to have inflammation defense reactions to all kind of normal foods. Fruits and grains can be a major instigator of a Crohn's flair up.

Sometimes the body is fine, and then sometimes not so much. Crohn's flair ups consist of abdominal and rectal pain. They can include irregular bowel movements, vomiting, and severe, incapacitating discomfort. A lot of people with Crohn's disease are on medications, have to be very careful about what they eat and the quality of food.

In severe cases, portions of the intestines need to be cut out. There are other surgeries that are meant to relieve Crohn's disease symptoms as well.

Since autoimmune diseases result in an imbalance in the body where the brain, immune system, and the target of the disease aren't communicating properly, Reiki energy is a great healing tool that can help correct the imbalance. It can also help with the physical pain from Crohn's disease.

Some people suffering from Crohn's disease have received Reiki sessions and been able to consume foods that they are otherwise not able to without the ordinary painful results. In other instances, Reiki can provide enough pain relief for people with Crohn's disease to get through their day or week without having to leave work or throw up or any of those other awful symptoms.

Any kind of disease that doesn't have a cure, that the surgeries aren't one hundred percent effective, or that can completely disrupt someone's life do take an emotional toll. Reiki is an asset to helping with the emotional and spiritual realignment. As in the case with any disease or illness, when the mind and spirit are aligned, the body can help itself better because it has less to focus on.

Surgical Recovery

Surgeries can be beneficial for lots of reasons. Surgeries can remove tumors, mend broken bones and joints, and relieve pressure that might otherwise cause death. Surgeries save lives with joint replacements and organ transplants.

Unless you have gone through a major surgery yourself, what you might not know is that the recovery process for surgery goes far beyond the physical recovery. Reiki energy is a noninvasive healing method that can be used immediately after a surgical procedure to help boost the immune system and speed up the recovery process.

Most therapies like massage and physical therapy require at least six weeks of healing before they can be used on a surgical patient. This is one reason Reiki is set apart from other healing methods.

Some surgical recoveries are so long that it can lead to other physical side effects like joint stiffness, atrophied muscles, and problems with scar tissue and surrounding connective tissues. Reiki can help keep the body balanced during recovery an minimize those side effects.

On an emotional level, some surgical recoveries are intense. Getting a joint replaced means having to adjust to that new joint. Having a limp amputated and getting a prosthetic is a whole other learning process. These can become frustrating and discouraging and even have addition painful side effects like phantom limb syndrome. Reiki can be used to ease the recovery process on an emotional level as well and has been successful in aiding with phantom limb syndrome in veterans.

Anyone who has gone through an organ transplant probably has friends who needed the same organ from a support group that didn't survive. This can lead to survivor's guilt and many other emotional complications. Again, Reiki can help relieve those emotional symptoms so the body can focus on healing. Reiki can also help the body adjust to and accept a new organ and lower the risks of rejection.

Chapter Nine:
Mental, Emotional and Spiritual Healing

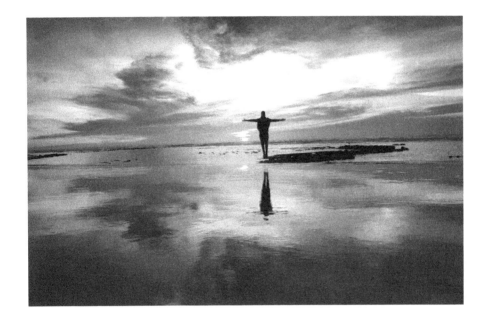

"The stiller you are, the calmer life is."
- Rasheed Ogunlaru

Sometimes ailments of the mind, emotional body, and spirit can be more debilitating than physical ailments. There are a few reasons for this. The first reason is that when the mind, emotions, and spirit are impacted it is usually an invisible pain that can't be measured by doctors and tools and can't visibly be seen by anyone else.

Unfortunately, this can lead to stigmas and unfair accusations that the pain isn't real or that the sufferer is making it up for attention or any other reason. Being in the position where this is the perception that others have of you can only add to the turmoil and the disease that impacts your mind, emotions, and spirit.

Sometimes these ailments can stem from a physical trauma, like physical abuse, but the lasting effects are mental, emotional, or spiritual. The physical body is just one layer in what makes a person. The western medical field has a strong focus on the physical body. This isn't necessarily a bad thing; however, it leaves the rest of the layers unnoticed and treats them as unimportant.

As more awareness about the different layers of people i.e. the emotional body and spiritual body, begins to grow and spread, disciplines like Reiki are becoming more popular and renowned. This is because therapies like Reiki have been used as a holistic healing method for centuries and Reiki does address all the different layers that can be impacted by imbalance and dis-ease.

When it comes to self-healing and personal power, having Reiki in your pocket as a tool that can be used is going to change the world for you. You'll have the ability make personal changes and shifts that may have seemed out of reach before. More than that, you'll have the ability to help yourself, even if no one else understands your suffering or thinks your suffering is real.

The truth is, everyone suffers, that is how change happens. Everyone experiences negativity, that is how they grow. With Reiki, you have the opportunity to help yourself and help others change and grow.

Some common ailments of the mind, emotional body, and spirit include:

- Depression
- Anxiety disorders
- Eating disorders
- Grief
- Anger Management
- Control issues

- OCD (Obsessive Compulsive Disorder)

While the severity of these ailments can vary greatly, anyone who has struggled with these ailments knows that the degree doesn't matter when you are trapped in the pattern that your mind creates around these symptoms.

Depression

Depression is classified as a lack of dopamine and serotonin production in the brain. It is a chemical imbalance that leads to feelings of sadness, dread, fear, paranoia, feeling stuck, having a lack of self-worth, lack of self-love, having low energy and no motivation.

Some cases of depression are so severe that people won't get out of bed for days, or their appetite vanishes and if no one reminds them to eat they become very malnourished. Depression can be debilitating and contribute to anxiety and paranoia preventing people from being able to leave their homes.

In some cases, being severely depressed leads to self-harming tendencies and suicide. The common treatment for depression is medication and psychotherapy.

Depression can be a result of trauma, abuse, or genetics. Sometimes there is no discernable reason.

Thankfully, awareness of mental health conditions like depression is growing. However, many people are still looking to alternative therapies such as Reiki to help with their depression. Medications can have side effects and most shouldn't be continued long term. Generally, people who are depressed are on more than one medication to stabilize themselves.

Reiki offers a noninvasive, nonpharmaceutical option to helping with depression symptoms. Reiki has been known to boost energy levels, increase motivation, and release energy related to traumas. Even if Reiki just opens the door to changes, like being able to take a walk every day, then the mind and body can begin healing the rest. It is the change from Reiki that allows you to take the next step in healing.

Anxiety Disorders
As with depression, awareness around anxiety disorders is becoming more prevalent and accepted. Anxiety disorders create an intense feeling of fear and worry within a person based on specific situations and

circumstances. This fear and worry can result in trouble sleeping, hyperventilating, panic attacks, sweating, and physical illness. In more severe cases, anxiety can become a phobia.

Some phobias and anxieties are so severe that people can't leave their own homes. Many people with severe anxieties and phobias are treated through talk therapy and medications.

This is why Reiki is so beneficial, because it can be sent over time and space. If someone is too anxious to leave their homes, Reiki can be sent to them to help balance their dis-ease and relieve their anxieties. Additionally, if you have anxety over social engagements, you can send Reiki to the time and place that you are engaging in a social activity. When you get there, the Reiki energy will be waiting for you to help ease your symptoms.

Grief
Grief is a deep-rooted sadness that stems from trauma, usually a loss of some kind. While it isn't the same as depression and it is more debilitating than regular sadness, grief can still disrupt everyday life.

When someone loses a loved one, family member, child, or pet, grief can become all consuming and they might not be able to move on. Letting go and moving on is the hardest part!

Reiki energy healing is all about releasing unneeded and unwanted energies, releasing imbalances and restoring balance. This is what makes it so effective in treating emotional imbalances such as excessive grief.

A certain amount of grief is healthy when it comes to loss. Excessive grief becomes the inability to move on, and that is when Reiki can become an asset.

Anger Management

Anger issues stem from a place of feeling powerless and out of control. There are different degrees of anger issues, some are more explosive and can even become violent. Part of the presentation of anger issues comes from society imposing the idea that all anger is bad and shouldn't be expressed.

When it doesn't get expressed, anger gets stored and becomes more and more dangerous for the person bottling it up and for the people around them. Most of the time, anger management issues are treated with talk therapy, support groups, and sometimes medication like mood stabilizers.

Reiki has a calming effect on the mind, body, and spirit. It creates a deep feeling of relaxation and also releases stored and blocked energies. If anger is something you struggle with, Reiki can help release what is stored, and the five Reiki principles can help you to change the way your mind and body react to potential anger in sighting situations.

Control Issues

Control issues are another ailment that originates from a place of feeling out of control or a lack of power. Control issues can manifest in many ways. Some people with control issues become meticulous and have to control every fine detail of their personal lives. Other people with control issues project them outward and start to micromanage the people around them.

From an energetic standpoint, control issues arise from an energetic imbalance in the solar plexus chakra. Reiki can help by balancing the solar plexus chakra, but Reiki helps in other ways as well. Through Gassho meditations you can learn to release and let go of that need for control. Reiki also increases your personal power and personal vibration, this essentially removes the lack of power feeling that creates a control issue.

OCD (Obsessive Compulsive Disorder)

OCD is a more prominent, severe kind of control disorder. The degrees of OCD vary and can be quite disruptive to everyday life. There is some evidence to suggest that OCD is a disorder where the brain doesn't have proper communication between various lobes. Treatment for OCD can be talk therapy and medication.

Unlike other disorders, depending on how severe OCD manifests, rationalization and logic can't override the OCD compulsions. The compulsions that manifest are often so programmed into the mind, and are a direct response to the way the brain communicates with the body, they become as natural and unconscious as your knee kicking out during a reflex test at the doctor's office. If a compulsive behavior isn't acted on, it creates a severe amount of anxiety within the person.

Reiki can greatly help reduce the symptoms of OCD which often include anxiety, paranoia, and phobias. Reiki can help with imbalances in the brain that might lead to OCD tendencies and compulsions. It can also release the energies that might be contributing to the compulsions.

As you can see, Reiki has so many uses when it comes to treating physical, mental, emotional, and spiritual ailments. Sometimes having it as a complimentary therapy to relieve symptoms is the best option. Other times, using it as a main treatment option yields the best results. Reiki is holistic and noninvasive and can be used in conjunction with medical treatments.

Self-Reiki treatments are going to be the best way for you to implement Reiki as a self-healing technique. There are other ways to utilize Reiki though, especially when it comes to mental, emotional, and spiritual healing. Meditation is going to be greatly beneficial to mental, emotional, and spiritual health. Reiki can be used in conjunction with meditation to achieve these goals.

To include Reiki in meditation, you can start or end your meditation with Gassho. You can perform your self-Reiki treatment before or after your meditation, or you can perform a meditation that directly incorporates Reiki into the process.

When you meditate, you'll want to find a quiet, secluded place where you can be alone and undisturbed for the duration of the meditation. You can make this space as relaxing and comfortable as you want, but be wary of falling asleep. Guided meditations are a great way to learn how to meditate if you are new to meditation.

Included in this chapter is a meditation exercise that is going to help you connect with Reiki energy and help you connect to your mind and spirit. This meditation will provide you with healing energy for the mind, emotions, and the spirit.

Meditation Exercise

- Find a quiet, relaxing place where you can be alone and undisturbed. Sit down comfortably and close your eyes. Ask that you be open to receiving Reiki energy.
- Take a deep breath in through your nose and out through our mouth. Feel the Reiki energy flowing though you. Breathe in deeply through your nose to the count of four and out through your mouth to

the count of eight. Breathe in through the nose to the count of four and out through your mouth to the count of eight.
- Continue to breathe deeply in through your nose and out through your mouth. Bring your hands together in the prayer position, your fingers touching and your palms spaced apart slightly.
- Hold your hands about four inches from your body and have the tips of your fingers pointing towards the sky, level with your brow or nose.
- In your third eye chakra, visualize the tips of your middle fingers with a bead of light at the top. Continue to breathe deeply in through the nose to the count of four and out through the mouth to the count of eight.
- Hold that bead of light in your third eye chakra.
- When you are called to, open your eyes and focus your attention on you're the tips of your middle fingers. Continue to breathe deeply in through your nose and out through your mouth. Set your focus to the tips of your middle fingers and if your mind begins to wander, refocus by pressing your middle fingers together.

- Continue to focus on your middle fingers with your eyes open, breathing deeply in through the nose and out through mouth.
- Close your eyes again and lower your hands into your lap. Take a deep breath in through the nose to the count of four and out through the mouth to the count of eight. Feel the Reiki energy in your hands. Perhaps your palms will feel warm or they will tingle with energy.
- Keeping your eyes closed, raise your dominant hand and place your fingers against your third eye chakra at your brow and feel the connection between Reiki and your third eye.
- Take another deep breath in through the nose and out through the mouth, lowing your fingers to your heart chakra at your sternum. Root the Reiki energy into your heart chakra before bringing your dominant hand back to your lap.
- Breathe deeply in through the nose to the count of four and out through the mouth to the count of eight.
- Raising your dominant hand again to the third eye chakra at your brow, place your fingers against your brow and breath deeply in through the nose and out through the mouth. Now bring your

dominant hand up to your crown chakra and lay your palm flat against the top of your head. Breath Reiki energy into your crown chakra and feel the connection there.
- Take a deep breath in through the nose to the count of four and out through the mouth to the count of eight.
- Bring your hand back to your heart chakra and root the Reiki energy into your heart center. Then release your hand back to your lap and continue to breathe deeply in through the nose and out through the mouth.
- In your mind's eye, visualize your crown chakra opening up to the cosmic universe and Reiki energy. Breathe in through your nose, drawing energy down through your crown chakra. Breathe out through the mouth to the count of eight. Breathe in again through your crown chakra, drawing Reiki energy down your spine and into the third eye chakra, throat chakra, heart chakra, solar plexus chakra, sacral chakra, and root chakra.
- Let the Reiki energy release with your exhale out the root chakra down towards your feet.
- Breathe in deeply through the crown chakra, drawing Reiki from the universe, through the crown

and down the spine to the third eye chakra, throat chakra, heat chakra, solar plexus chakra, sacral chakra, and root chakra.
- Breathe out through the mouth, releasing Reiki energy out of the root chakra and out towards the feet.
- Take a deep breath in through the nose to the count of four and out through the mouth to the count of eight. Start to come back to your physical body. Breathe in through the nose and out through the mouth, connecting back to your skin. Breathe in through the nose and out through the mouth.
- When you have completed your meditation, perform a grounding exercise if necessary.

Chapter Ten:
Reiki Level I and II

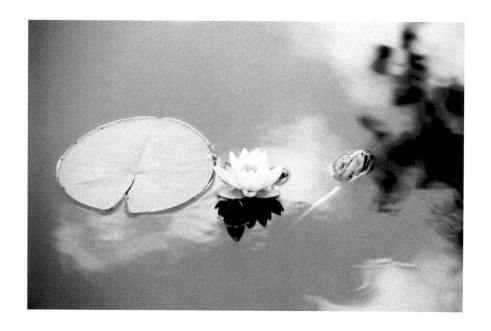

"Many people are alive, but don't touch the miracle of being alive."
- *Thich Nhat Hanh*

In the first chapter of this book, the different levels of Reiki were discussed and broken down into degrees. In traditional Usui Reiki there are three levels, which in the western teachings are referred to as Reiki Level I, Reiki Level II, and Reiki Master Level. Each level teachings different concepts and uses of Reiki and attunes you to different aspects of Reiki.

If your intention is to only use Reiki for yourself and sometimes friends and family, then Reiki Level I is the basic level that would meet your needs. However, if you intend to use Reiki professionally and as a paid service, it is recommended that you learn at least Reiki Level II because you will be attuned to the Reiki power symbols and that will greatly enhance your healing sessions. The Reiki Master level is often for advanced Reiki techniques and to attune you with the wisdom of teaching other Reiki students and attuning them to Reiki.

There are some fundamental differences between Reiki level I and Reiki Level II when it comes to learning and attunements. By reviewing the differences, hopefully you will be able to better determine the best learning path for yourself.

That being said, you don't have to learn all the Reiki levels at once. You don't have decide now how far you want to go. You can always decide later that you'd like to progress further in your studies as things change. Right now, discussing the differences between Reiki Level I and Reiki Level II is going to help you determine where you should be in your studies and what you want to gain from your studies.

Reiki Level I

In Reiki Level I you learn the basics. This doesn't mean that you have to learn beyond Reiki Level I to be a successful Reiki practitioner. Think of it like college degrees. There are Associate Degrees, Bachelor Degrees, Masters Degrees, and PhD's. Each degree level brings you a deeper understanding of the subject material.

This is the same with Reiki levels. There are millions of people in the world that are successful and happy with an Associates Degree and never feel the need to take their education beyond that point. So it is with Reiki Level I, thousands of practitioners learn Reiki Level I and never need to or want to move further.

What do you learn in Reiki Level I? Reiki Level I course material often includes a comprehensive history of Reiki. This includes legends and myths, historical data, and information on how Reiki spread and expanded through the world. You'll learn about the founders of Reiki and how they changed the way it was taught and performed.

You will be taught about energy and what Reiki energy is, how it works, and how the body responds to it. You'll also be taught about energetic anatomy and physical anatomy and how Reiki is beneficial to holistic healing. You might even learn about specific ailments, illnesses, and diseases that can benefit from Reiki energy healing.

In Reiki Level I you learn about the five Reiki principles and how to incorporate them into your life, meditations, and Reiki practices. In learning about the Reiki principles, you'll also learn about energy and how shifts in your own energy and person life can change your entire world.

Reiki Level I courses will discuss different applications of Reiki, such as prenatal care, palliative care, group sessions, and provide resources to further your Reiki education. Prenatal care, child, and infant care is working with pregnant women, infants, and mothers and children. Palliative care is working with seniors and the elder. Group sessions are performed when multiple practitioners work on a single recipient.

The point of including these different types of Reiki sessions and uses of Reiki energy is to help you discover what you can do with Reiki. Know its benefits and uses will guide you to how you want to use Reiki and possibly lead you to a niche or specialty in your Reiki practice.

Since Reiki Level I isn't just an introductory course to what Reiki is, you'll also learn about self-Reiki treatments and treating others with Reiki. Through this part of the course you will learn the hand positions for a self-treatment and the hand positions to use when treating others.

Not only you will learn the hand positions, but your Reiki Master should also provide you with detailed information on how to setup and prepare for performing Reiki sessions, on yourself and others. They should teach you about the limitations of Reiki when it comes to prescribing and diagnosing, working with someone else's aura and chakras, and the steps of performing a session on someone else. This will include how to greet and talk to a client when you first meet them and what should be discussed when the session is over.

If you are taking an in-person course, you should have the opportunity to practice these hand positions hands on with other students or with your Reiki Master. If you are taking an online course, there will most likely be an assignment that requires you to practice a certain number of self-Reiki sessions and Reiki sessions on someone else.

Most Masters will incorporate mediations into their Reiki Level I courses. They will emphasize the importance of daily self-treatments and daily meditation. You may even be given mediation exercises to practice and complete.

Reiki Level I is the door into the world of energy, personal growth, and self-discovery. This level is going to be more focused on how you can benefit from Reiki and how you can use Reiki in your personal life. You'll learn about using Reiki on food and drink and in other daily applications that you might not think to use Reiki in.

Every Reiki Master teaches their courses a little differently. However, these are the common basics that are covered in Reiki Level I courses.

The knowledge you gain from a Reiki Level I course gives you everything you need to succeed in using Reiki to shift your personal energies, align yourself, and raise your own energy to your highest vibration.

Reiki Level II

Reiki Level II courses become more in-depth with what is taught and learned. A Reiki Level II course should include a small review of what was learned in Reiki Level I, just to ensure everyone is on the same page.

By the time you reach Reiki Level II, you should have enough preliminary knowledge to know where you'd like to take your Reiki studies and how you plan to apply your knowledge. Whether this is in starting a Reiki practice to heal others, focusing on improving your own life, health, and wellness, or just branching out in the Reiki community to meet new people and gain new experiences. Level II Reiki is going to give you the knowledge and wisdom to take your studies and healing to the next level.

One of the biggest differences in Reiki level I and Reiki Level II is the Reiki power symbols. These power symbols are taught at the Level II degree and then your Master will attune you to them at the Level II degree.

There are three Reiki power symbols that are included in the Reiki Level II course. These symbols have different meanings and uses and expand your ability to use and apply Reiki healing energy to different situations.

The first Reiki power symbol is Cho-Ku-Rei or CKR. Cho Ku Rei means: placing the power of the universe here." It is an amplification symbol that is meant to increase the potency of Reiki energy. The below picture outlines what the Cho Ku Rei symbol looks like and how to draw it.

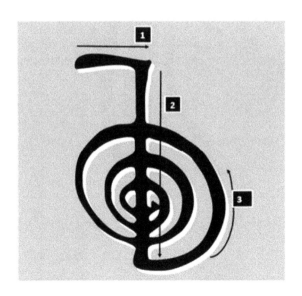

The second symbol that is taught in Reiki Level II is Sei-He-Ki or SHK symbol. This is the emotional healing symbol and is very powerful when treating people, or yourself, for any emotional troubles. The translation of this symbol means: The earth and sky meet or become one. It is a balancing symbol.

The following picture is what the Sei He Ki symbol looks like and how it should be drawn.

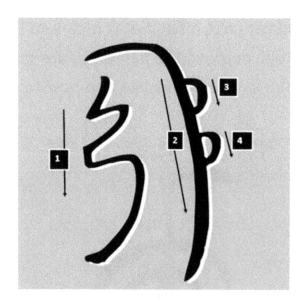

The third Reiki power symbol that is taught at Reiki Level II is the Hon-Sha-Ze-Sho-Nen or HSZSN symbol. Hon Sha Ze Sho Nen is the distance symbol that can send Reiki over time and space. It means: having no past, present, or future. Hon Sha Ze Sho Nen is depicted in the picture below with a diagram of how it should be drawn.

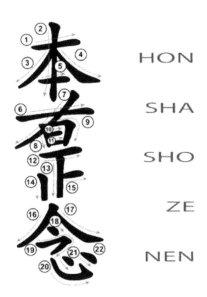

These three power symbols greatly enhance Reiki healing sessions and deepen your connection to Reiki energy. In a Reiki Level II course, you'll learn about how to properly intone and activate the symbols as well as the different applications for them.

Once you understand the meanings behind the power symbols, your use of Reiki is going to greatly advance. Reiki power symbols can be used directly on the body. They can be used in a room or space. With the HSZSN symbol, you can beam Reiki energy and Reiki power symbols to s specific time, place, or situation.

The power symbols can be infused into items like food and water, clothing, jewelry, even electronics.

Once you learnt he power symbols and their uses, you'll also learn about the three pillars or Reiki. While the pillars can be adapted to use without the Reiki power symbols, they are designed to primarily include the Reiki power symbols as part of the process.

Between the Reiki power symbols and the three pillars or Reiki you'll already have a much more profound connection and understanding of this energy.

If you are taking an in-person course, you should have the opportunity to practice using, intoning, and drawing the three Reiki power symbols on another student or on your teacher. You should also get the chance to practice the three pillars of Reiki in a treatment session on another student or on your teacher.

For an online course, you'll probably be given an assignment such as drawing each Reiki power symbol twice a day, or performing five sessions with the Reiki power symbols, or even performing five distance Reiki sessions.

At this level, you'll learn deeper Reiki techniques like how to perform distance Reiki sessions, how Reiki can be used to heal past traumas and past lives. You'll learn about sending Reiki to a time and place, or a situation that hasn't happened yet. This is going to expand on how and when you are able to perform Reiki sessions for yourself and others.

Often times, Reiki Level II is when you will be introduced to some Advanced Reiki Techniques. This might include performing Reiki sessions on animals. Animals benefit from Reiki healing energy just as profoundly as humans do. If you ever have doubts about energy work, perform a Reiki session on an animal.

Animals are so intuitive about their bodies and their needs. They are also far more sensitive to the energy naturally. People often have to work towards being sensitive to energy by developing their intuition and through meditation and receiving and performing Reiki sessions. Animals are already connected to their intuition and their energy senses.

This means that they will often display more drastic physical, emotional, and behavioral reactions to Reiki energy during a session. Many people who have been skeptical about Reiki have witnessed a session performed on an animal and afterwards have professed without a doubt that they witnessed something happening with the animal.

If you do get the opportunity to learn Reiki for Animals, working with animals is highly rewarding and also very therapeutic work.

Another advanced Reiki technique that might be introduced at the Reiki Level II degree is Crystal Reiki. In a Crystal Reiki course, you learn about the properties and energetic power of crystals. You also learn about the application of crystals in Reiki relating to the chakras. There are various methods for activating crystal energy in a Reiki session, including crystal grids.

Learning about the energy of geometric shapes and crystal grids brings you a whole new set of tools for using

Reiki for healing. Crystal work in Reiki has the benefit of allowing you to focus the energy and intention of your session more specifically than a traditional Reiki session.

Reiki Level II is going to focus more on how you can enhance sessions when practicing on other people. This is why it is recommended that you take up to Reiki Level II if you plan on using Reiki healing as a professional healing service.

There will also be more focus on including Reiki into daily practices such as meditation, or infusing items and object with Reiki to use personally on your path to health and wellness.

As with Reiki Level I courses, each Master is going to teach their Reiki Level II course a little differently. The Reiki power symbols and the three pillars of Reiki are the primary difference between Reiki Level I and Reiki Level II.

In Reiki Level II you learned about self-treatment sessions and performing Reiki sessions on others. You also learned about the five pillars of Reiki and the best ways to incorporate Reiki into your life. In Reiki Level II you will learn about the Reiki power symbols and three pillars or Reiki. You will expand and deepen your knowledge on Reiki energy and how to heal yourself, others, and apply it to daily life.

Chapter Eleven:
Other Reiki Applications

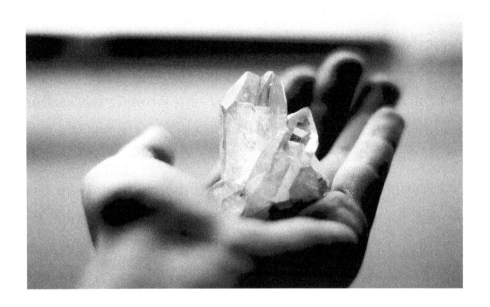

"You are the sky. Everything else is just the weather."
- Pema Chodron

Reiki energy healing is versatile. It isn't just beneficial in self-treatments or in healing others. Reiki can be applied to mundane, simple, everyday tasks and actions that you do regardless of what changes and shifts you make in your life. Reiki has the power to enhance every task, action and experience throughout your day.

You might find it excessive to include Reiki in every moment of your day. Or, you might find it absolutely wonderful to include Reiki into every moment and task of your day. The more you use Reiki, the more you will find uses for it. You will also find how and when it works best for you.

For example, if you have a job interview coming up that you are feeling anxious or nervous about, try using the HSZSN symbol to send Reiki to the time and place of your job interview. This can certainly help you relax and benefit the outcome of the job interview. If you aren't attuned to Reiki level II and the power symbols, you can perform a quick five to ten-minute Reiki session on yourself prior to the job interview to help settle your nerves and relax yourself. By bringing yourself into a balanced, harmonious state, the job interview will go much smoother.

Job interviews aren't every day occurrences, unless you are actively looking for a job. While they are a part of adulthood in most cases, using Reiki in a job interview is more of a specialized example. There are daily tasks and actions that can benefit from Reiki as well. Eating food and drinking water or beverages is a daily action. People need to drink and eat to survive. Reiki can benefit food and drink consumption.

Exercise should be a part of daily life. Reiki can benefit you as you exercise and can also provide you with the motivation and energy to begin an exercise routine.

You might find that if you and your spouse or partner aren't seeing eye to eye, by sending Reiki to the time and place of your interactions can help ease the tension. You could also use Reiki in the rooms of your house to clear out any negative energies that can be contributing to the tension you are feeling with your spouse or partner.

Sometimes an argument can linger longer than it should, feeding animosity and discomfort in the home. Using Reiki on a specific situation, argument, or disagreement by sending Reiki directly to that situation, even if it is in the past, can help bring you and your spouse or partner clarity on the situation and also provide you with a resolution.

The balancing and healing qualities of Reiki go beyond just healing sessions. Because Reiki heals and balances, when energies are aligned and shifted into balance this opens the mind and perception up to clarity. Often times, having clarity on a matter will then guide you to a balanced, civil resolution.

Reiki with Food and Drink

To use Reiki in food or drink, you can simply hold your hands around a cup, plate, bowl, or food receptacle and ask that Reiki energy flow through you into your food or drink.

If you are attuned to Reiki Level II, drawing and activating the Reiki power symbols over your food or drink, or on the container they are in, will also infuse that food or drink item with Reiki energy.

Why infuse food and drink with Reiki? Several reasons. First of all, the amount of energies your food comes into contact with from where it is grown or raised to when it is harvested, processed, packaged, and shelved is vast. Your food can pickup traces of all those energies, some are negative, some aren't. Using Reiki on your food and drink helps to clear it of those energies and ensure that you are only consuming the energies that align with your highest vibration.

Another reason to infuse food and drink with Reiki could be that you have an eating disorder or are prone to emotional eating, or maybe when you get stressed you lose your appetite for days. These are strong emotional responses to imbalances in the body. However, infusing food and drink with Reiki energy can help the consumption and digestion of food and help you create a healthy connection with food and eating again.

Food and drink are sources of nourishment. This means that they are a basic fundamental need to survival. Don't underestimate the value of having a strong connection to your food and drink as a source of your nourishment and life force. Reiki can help provide with that connection to your food.

Reiki with Exercise

The human body is designed to move and stay active in order to stay healthy and functional. Humans evolved as hunter gatherers. This means that a great portion of their time involved following herds of animals on foot, being out in the wilderness hunting wild game and gathering berries, roots, and other food sources.

The body evolved to sustain endurance running, deep breathing, and a large range of motion with over three hundred joints in the body.

In modern society where humans no longer have to hunt and gather, especially in the age of technology where so much happens at a computer screen, television, or smart phone screen, the idea of movement and exercise gets put on the back burner for a lot of people. Unfortunately, this can lead to weight gain, increases in blood pressure and cholesterol, atrophied muscles, stiff joints, fluid build up in the joints, neuropathy, and many other easily avoidable conditions and imbalances in the body.

By making exercise and movement a regular part of your routine, your body maintains a much more physically, mentally, and spiritually healthy state. Sometimes it is hard to exercise though. The energy output for a full-time job reduces the energy that you might have to apply to exercise. This is true for the energy it takes to raise a family and keep a house as well.

Having a lack of energy or a lack of motivation can become a huge crutch when it comes to exercise. Fortunately, Reiki can help. Put your exercise clothes on and then do a quick Reiki session, holding your hands on your legs, arms, and chest. Then go out for a quick walk. Maybe start by just doing the quick sessions on yourself without following the session with exercise. Eventually, you will feel compelled to follow up with exercise and you'll have the energy and motivation to do it.

Some people use exercise as a way to lose weight or maintain weight. Reiki can assist in this process as well. By using Reiki symbols on the areas of your body that you want to target for weight loss before a workout can help amplify the effects of the exercise and Reiki energy to that area of the body.

If you aren't attuned to Reiki Level II, just placing your hands on a target around and performing a quick five-minute Reiki session will also help to target that area during your workout.

Reiki in the Home
There are many instances around the house where you can come to find Reiki as beneficial. Some of those

instances could involve a spouse or partner. Other times, they might be in regard to personal situations. For example, having the motivation and energy to complete chores around the house can be enhanced with Reiki energy on yourself or by sending it to the situation in which you find you need it.

If you haven't folded the laundry in three days but it is dry and sitting in the basket, ask Reiki to flow through you and send it to the task of folding laundry. If you are attuned to Reiki Level II, use the Reiki power symbols on yourself or on the laundry basket to help align your motivation and energy with the task of folding laundry.

Maybe you haven't been able to focus on something like paying bills, writing a letter, or drawing a picture. Reiki can be used for personal hobbies as well, like art and do it yourself projects. Maybe you started knitting a sweater and haven't been able to focus enough to finish it.

Send Reiki into the knitting needles, the yarn, and into the part of the project that has been finished. Use Reiki on your head, your throat chakra, your sacral chakra, and your hands to help stimulate the creativity and focus that will go into finishing your knitting project.

There are many instances of physical activities or emotional situations that you can find Reiki to be helpful around the house. Whether it is with chores, personal hobbies and projects, or with the relationships you have with the other members of your household, you can apply Reiki to benefit these situations and tasks.

It can take some practice to start using Reiki in these situations, but your intuition will help you and the more you do it, the more fluid and natural it will start to feel.

Reiki and Crystals
Along with daily activities and task, Reiki can be combined with other health and wellness practices and modalities to enhance your healing experience and further increase your energetic vibration.

Crystals are another tool that has been utilized in healing for centuries, but fell out of favor in the middle ages with the modernization of science and western medicine. Since alternative therapies are coming back into practice, crystals are starting to get more attention and more focus again.

On their own, crystals are an incredibly powerful source of natural energy. They are also one of the most stable forms of matter to occur naturally. These qualities mean that crystals can transform, absorb, refract, reflect, store, and transmute energy, including energy in the human body.

Every crystal has a set of properties that coincide with how they were formed, their color, their internal geometric crystalline structure, and the frequency of energy that they vibrate at. These properties and qualities react to and benefit the body on a physical, emotional, and spiritual level. Crystals are natural amplifiers of energy as well.

Crystals can benefit a Reiki session by amplifying the Reiki energy. More than that, because crystals have specific properties, they can be used to focus Reiki energy for a more specific purpose and task in a healing session. If you are interested in working with crystals with Reiki, it is an advanced Reiki technique that requires additional attunements and study, but the combination of Reiki and crystals is powerful. Crystals are another healing tool that you can use on yourself.

For more information on crystal healing, properties, and crystals with Reiki, make sure to check out *Crystals Healing for Beginners* as part of this series.

Reiki and Meditation

Meditation is another health and wellness practice. It should also become a part of your daily routine. Meditation is about relaxing and calming the mind. The goal isn't to let go of your thoughts and clear your head completely, the goal is to keep your thoughts from controlling you.

Through meditation you can retrain your brain and body to react and think differently in ways that will ultimate raise your vibration and lead to a fulfilling, successful life. For over two thousand years mediation has been incorporated into spiritual ceremonies, rites of passage, and religious teachings. Many spiritual and religious practitioners today still take intense mediation journeys.

When done properly, meditation can actually alter the state of consciousness that the mind is in. What this means is that meditation can alter the brain waves, bringing them to the Theta Brain Wave level which is somewhere between Delta Waves, which are sleep waves, and Beta Waves, which are relaxing and rejuvenating waves. When the mind reaches Theta waves it enters into a trancelike state where you can truly connect to spirit and the cosmic energies of the universe.

Reiki can assist with meditation in the form of Gassho. You can also begin a meditation with a quick Reiki session, or intoning some of the Reiki power symbols if you are attuned. Reiki combined with meditation can open you up to a deeper spiritual experience but also provide you with a broader wisdom and understanding of yourself. Through this process you can truly discover yourself and the right path for you to follow in your pursuit of health and wellness.

Appendix A

This book, *Reiki Healing for Beginners*, one of three books in a complete series for healing, personal power, mindfulness, and raising your energetic vibration. Individually, the books have great information, knowledge and wisdom to guide you. Together, all three books make a comprehensive guide to discovering yourself and living your most fulfilling, successful life at the highest vibration you can.

The other two books in the series are *Crystals Healing for Beginners* and *Chakras Healing for Beginners.* Be sure to check them out as additions to your collection!

<u>Crystals Healing for Beginners</u> covers the uses and properties of crystals and their energy. With this book you can unlock the amazing, natural, energetic power of crystals and learn how to use them in your daily life. More than that, you will discover how crystals can be used with Reiki energy healing and how they can be used to heal the chakras. Individually crystals have amazing power, learn how to use it for your personal health, wellness, and personal power.

Chakras Healing for Beginners is an in-depth look at the energetic systems in your body. These are crucial systems that contribute to a lot of physical, emotional, and mental symptoms that create disruption in your life. By learning about the chakras, you can empower yourself to heal yourself and find balance in your life. You'll learn how to combine Reiki energy and crystals with your chakras and energy systems for a complete, holistic healing and balancing experience.

Conclusion

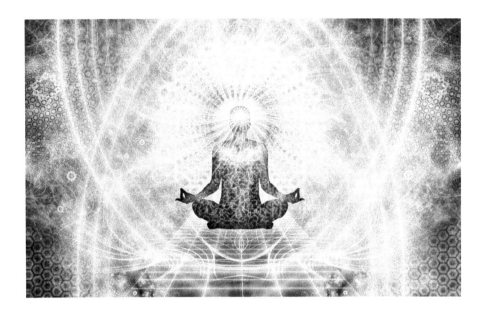

"You only lose what you cling to."
- *Buddha*

Thank you for making it through all the chapters of *Reiki Healing for Beginners.* Hopefully you found the information to be relevant and interesting. Now you should have the knowledge and guidance and tools you need to achieve your goals whatever they may be.

Now that you have completed this part of the series, the next step to take is to find a Reiki Master or practitioner. If you have not already done so, look for a practitioner that you resonate with so you can begin your Reiki Level I course. Make sure to find a practitioner who you feel comfortable with and one that you resonate with.

As you search for a Reiki Master, start making mediation practices a regular part of your daily routine. This is going to be the first step in clearing yourself and releasing unwanted energies so that when you receive your Reiki attunement ceremony, you'll be more open and aligned to those energies. If you can, make small shifts in your diet and lifestyle to help foster open energetic channels as you continue down this path of personal healing and personal empowerment.

Since the path you have chosen to walk is going to create shifts in your body, mind, spirit, and your physical environment, begin keeping a journal or notebook of your experiences. This is going to help you track the subtle shifts and changes, and also give you a way to reflect back on your progress.

Finally, if you found this book useful in any way, a review on Amazon is always appreciated! Don't forget to check out the other books in this series *Crystals Healing for Beginners* and *Chakras Healing for Beginners* for the complete set.

Karen.

CPSIA information can be obtained
at www.ICGtesting.com
Printed in the USA
LVHW051438270420
654512LV00019B/2437